MONSTER BRAIN

Titles Available from
Forty-Two Books

Peaks of Madness: A Collection of Utah Horror

Strange Stories Volume 1

Satan Speaks! Contemporary Satanic Voices

Putrescent Poems Volume 1

The Dress: A Poetic Response

They Walk Among Us: A Collection of Utah Horror

All Titles Available on Amazon.com or from Forty-Two Books

MONSTER BRAIN
Conversations with OCD

Poems and Writings by

Daniel Cureton

42 Books
Salt Lake City

Copyright © 2019. All rights reserved.
A Forty-Two Books, LLC. original publication,
Salt Lake City, UT, USA.
Printed in USA on acid free paper.

ISBN-13: 978-1-7340067-3-5
LCCN: 2019913981

Forty-Two Books, LLC maintains exclusive rights over the works contained in this volume. Reproduction, transmission, photocopying, scanning, and other dissemination of works contained within in print, audio, or digital form (outside of personal and scholastic study) is prohibited. For permissions, please contact the publisher.

Cover Art by Kapitosh—see "Bibliography, "images, licensed commercial usage" for full details, page 158.

Contact
Forty-Two Books, LLC.
P.O. Box 57474
Murray, UT 84157
USA
Email: info@fortytwobooks.com
Web: www.fortytwobooks.com

First Edition. Second Printing.
November 2020.

To The Silent Sufferers:
You are not alone.

ACKNOWLEDGMENTS

I want to thank all those who were there to support me in my time of need: April M. Love for the continued love, stability, and support; Darby Fanning for her hospitality and kinship; Sherelyn and Earl Cureton, my parents; Naomi Spencer for following her instincts; Cam James for helping me understand my new self; The OCD and Anxiety Center of Bountiful, UT; Aaron Ershlar for his friendship; and to all the friends I found I had through the struggle: Jazmin Chang, Deb Chittur, Kathryn Cottle, Alana Howlett, Jason Richy, and Barkingham's Brenda (of Tooele, UT).

INTRODUCTION

The day you break down comes like a hand in the dark. You're fine one moment, and broken the next. Unprepared, exposed, and completely at the mercy of those who can help you.

Monster Brain is a personal journey. My story, through understanding Obsessive Compulsive Disorder (or intrusive thought disorder as I call it), the road to healing, and finding life again as a changed man.

The majority of OCD sufferers suffer in silence. They are bombarded with intrusive thoughts, feelings, phantom emotions, thoughts fusing with sensations to feel real (thought-fused action), and other sensations which lead them to do a compulsion (like flipping the switch or checking a lock). Their own brain is telling them an emergency is under way. If they don't do the compulsion to ease the exponential increase in anxiety, something horrible will happen, such as their family dying. The compulsions ease the anxiety for a few moments, but the attacks come back, over and over, never ceasing.

Sufferers are *too* empathetic. Unlike the psychopath, when the undesired image bursts into the conscious mind frame, they can't let it float by as most people do. They analyze, they feel shame, anger, guilt, and ask themselves: "What kind of person am I to think such thoughts, I would never do such a thing" "Why am I thinking this, I don't want to be a criminal." and "God, why am I suffering, you know my heart is pure!" Their empathy makes them obsess over the meaning—they feel that they can tell no one.

Logic and reason doesn't work either to rid the intrusive thoughts; the rational brain knows something is wrong but can't help. They think that the thoughts of murder, pedophilia, contamination, or that they have run someone over in the street, means they are a terrible, unworthy, and an unlovable person.

But thoughts are thoughts. Until you act on them, they harm no one. They don't have to mean anything except being just garbage thoughts from some dark corner of your <u>non-conscious</u> brain.

OCD changes forms. Once a person has the lock checking under control for example, it'll shift from contamination and blaspheming, to loosing your mind, skin picking, or a whole host of other behaviors in an attempt to get the person to do compulsions. The compulsions are what feed <u>it</u>—OCD—giving in confirms the fear, and confirms the emergency, when in reality their never was one and you were perfectly safe.

Those who suffer try therapy and meds, and mostly can lead a normal life. They learn to manage the anxiety, depression, and compulsions. They recognize the OCD monster is trying to feed, but choose to starve it instead by *not* doing the compulsions.

This book begins at what I feel are earlier iterations of OCD in my life, then moves into the build up, the breakdown phase, and ends with the healing stage, woven with the experiences of other OCD sufferers.

All writings are original work composed after my diagnosis in 2019. Included is mostly poems but also flash fiction, film scripts, a play, and experimental pieces. This book is a mix because when I sat down to write, some of the narratives wouldn't have worked as a poem and I tried my best to convey my experience (my head space). The poems are in many different poetic forms such as haiku, sonnet, limerick, letters, idyll, epistolary, rhyme, pantoum, free verse, narrative, and villanelle.

I chose to transform my OCD into art, into writing, and poetry. To describe, in detail, the experiences for someone who never knew they suffered, but when they reflected back on their life and saw points where OCD was overshadowing them. While very

Daniel Cureton

personal, I decided the best way to beat the damn thing was to trick it: Expose the reality of what is it, how it operates, the mental space a person finds themselves.

May this book help you, help you know what OCD masquerades as, and to let you know that there is community—you do not have to sufferer in silence, and alone.

Daniel Cureton, MA
September 20, 2019,
Salt Lake City, UT, USA

MONSTER BRAIN

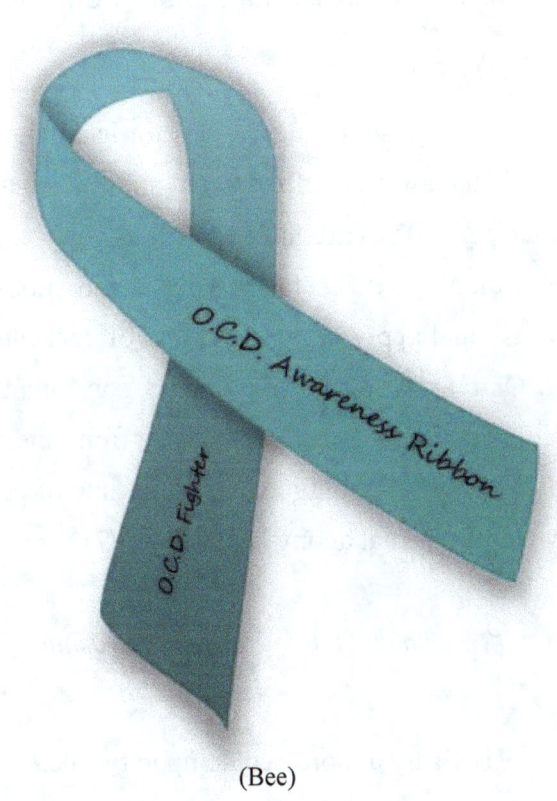

(Bee)

THE TENTH RULE

From the Handbook of the Militant Christian

"Tenth Rule

Here are some suggestions for handling temptation: Make a violent effort to put sinful thoughts out of your mind. Turn around and spit, as it were, in the face of the tempter. Or fasten your attention on some holy task and apply all your powers of concentration to it. Or pray with all your might. You might have some particularly stirring passages from the Bible ready to use to encourage yourself in time of particularly painful mental agony" (Erasmus, 77).

Pff, we know that doesn't work Erasmus!!

Let's try a more...contemporary rule.

MONSTER BRAIN
Cureton's Tenth Rule, Updated for the 21st Century

"*Tenth Rule*

Here are some suggestions for handling temptation or obsession: Make a peaceful effort to put unwanted thoughts out of your mind. Turn around and laugh, as it were, in the face of yourself. Or fasten your attention on some unholy task and apply all your powers of concentration to it. Or work magick with all your might. You might have some particularly stirring passages from *The Satanic Verses* ready to use to encourage yourself in time of particularly painful mental agony" (Cureton, 13).

You can find new stirring passages within:

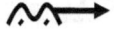

Daniel Cureton

PRESCRIBED CONVERSATIONS

Acknowledgements 6
Introduction 7
The Tenth Rule 12
Prescribed Conversations 14
Bibliography 155
About the Author 165

The Conversations

#SoOCD 19
Demons, Demons, Demons 26
Monsters are Real 28
Jizzus Christ: The Flasher 30
Perfection 32
My Best Ghost 34
Donatello 36
Deb 40
Heart of Terror 41
Anxiety's Bane 44
Fog 46
The Art of Breaking 48
Alone in a Crowd: A Short Film by OCD 58

MONSTER BRAIN

Intermountain Faeries 64
The Intake 67
Depression Riots 70
A Day in the Life of Compulsion 73
Naomi: 1 – OCD: 0 79
Pure-O 80
The Pose 82
The Man at the Counter Who Served Lunch 83
The Red Wall 84
Oh Brenda 86
My Nurses 87
To Have a Cam 88
White Pill: A Short Film 90
Note to Self 96
What Isn't Right: A Catalogue 97
The Blur 100
Fatigue 102
OCD Center 104
To Aaron 106
Dirty Diaper 108
Five Nights at Darby's 110
Brain Trippin' 113
Studio of Apollo 115
The Long, Long Shower 118
Hypochondriasis 120

Daniel Cureton

Let the Bodies Hit the Road 122
The Skin Picker 125
Heteroflexible? 126
Debussy's Idyll 128
Trichotillomania 132
That Damned Lock 134
Love the Children 136
Hand Washer: A One Scene Play 138
The Silent Sufferers 142
Hue of Blue 148
Through Fire, and Water 149
I Bid Adieu 151

"Control your emotions. Discipline your mind!"
—Severus Snape.

THE CONVERSATIONS

MONSTER BRAIN

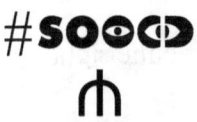

You just finished a deep clean
and turned all your book spines around.
You fill the waste bin
and fall flat onto the ground.

You open your Insta
and take a pic.
You type a simple message,
"I'm *#soOCD, LOL ^_^" click!*

You close the app,
"likes" guaranteed;
move through your day's work,
floating on potpourri.

Little did you know
what you really said;
commenting on a condition,
concerning the head.

Daniel Cureton

The brain is the enemy,
the monster inside,
that tells you, "it's not quite right,"
till you're begging to die.

Anxiety overwhelms
and panic sets the win,
as you can't control the compulsions
and find the time to fit them in.

Obsession isn't about cleaning,
organizing, or matching books,
but the discomfort that comes
from all the intrusive hooks.

The hours spent fighting
the anguished mental flip,
and the movements that bring relief
on OCD's eternal grip.

The loop repeats
and the anguish continues.
Lives wasted away
in obedience, retinues.

MONSTER BRAIN

Some are told "the germs will kill,"
their family will die
if they don't perform this
precise ritual—with no reason why.

"It just doesn't feel right
the way I pass the mirror."
So I walk back again
my own interferer.

They check the light switch,
knew it was turned off,
flip it up and down
till the skin is slowly doffed.

Others run from the knives
afraid in the kitchen.
The horror reels show them
Murderer become, fixin'.

The hetero man wakes up in the morning
carnal desires topic of the day
—forced on mind,
OCD screams he's gay.

Daniel Cureton

The Saint texts in the pew
as the prayer meeting ends.
All the voice says
is blasphemes to send.

Mom is so afraid of the sickening plagues
"My child will die, I'm out of wit.
oh god, he's caught a cough…
I know this is it!"

You will never have to feel
the long endless nights
as OCD victims suffer
from their own restless frights.

Brain that's gone wrong
organic machine collapsed.
No logic can reason it
and prevent the hours that will elapse.

No haunting voice
or pressing urges
consume your gentle soul
as you seek, the fear, to purges.

MONSTER BRAIN

Life to live for,
medication free.
No white pills,
no anxiety—no therapy.

So be glad,
OCD is nothing you really knew
just some books and cleaning,
throwing away the old you.

Daniel Cureton

DEMONS, DEMONS, DEMONS

Belial!
Behemoth!
Beelzebub!

On and on the loop rolls.
I can't break the cycle
as demon names take their tolls.

Asmodeus!
Satan!
Lucifer!

My Christian heart weeps in tears,
offended at the sounds
as my Jesus mind abandons me with a sneer.

Leviathan!
Mammon
Belphegor!

MONSTER BRAIN

Not the possession!
What did a good boy like me do
to deserve such an obsession?

Devil! *Lord of Flies!*
Chanting away, as the dark mass tells.
Satanic rites—passages born in night give sway to lies.

Why does this happen to a boy of the hood (priest),
when he prayed so much
and begged god as he stood.

Forgive the suckling—
the devil's nuts!

MONSTERS ARE REAL

It came through the door when I looked,
I didn't know what to do.
It was the blob monster,
without any shoes.

Johnny Quest flashed on the screen,
but I wasn't as bold.
Terrified of the image seen,
I was only 4 years old.

I closed my eyes tightly
To make it go away:
The image of the monster covered in paint,
to me, wending its way.

Burned, bludgeoned,
setting the village on fire.
I sat frightened of the shadows
of my mind's bog and ire.

MONSTER BRAIN

It was always in the dark bathroom
in the naval base housing.
Mother and father's room,
who knew nothing of my brain's lousing.

The organic machine,
so tired for the image on loop.
I couldn't make it go away,
not even while praying to Babadook.

Never leaving,
but hiding in plain sight.
The haunting image and my struggle
was anxiety's terrible fright.

What was child to do,
who knew nothing of the world,
except hide under the covers
and lie there furled.

Daniel Cureton

JIZZUS CHRIST: THE FLASHER

Some of my early memories of OCD
come from my teen years.
Sure, the occasional dream:
A blanket covering a very spikey object
"didn't feel right" when I was 6.

The instrusivity began early.
Orthodox Mormon
in the Deep South—
everything was religious—
we lived and breathed Faith.

We were surrounded by the boundless churches
on every corner.
Morning, noon, and night was Church.
Seminary, study, missionary dinners,
and night time prayers.

Mormon Jesus would slide into my brain—
gay flower budding—
Flashing the Sacred Masculine Meat!

MONSTER BRAIN

It was ever so clear—
never planned—
and came on his hands (much like Ra).
Dripping through the hole—
delicious divine cum—
breeding new life
in a southern boy's tum.

В꙳ *Flasher Jesus* ꙳Ω

Revealed of cloak,
showing me all of
the
Father,
The Son—
with which he,
made,
 t h e
universe…

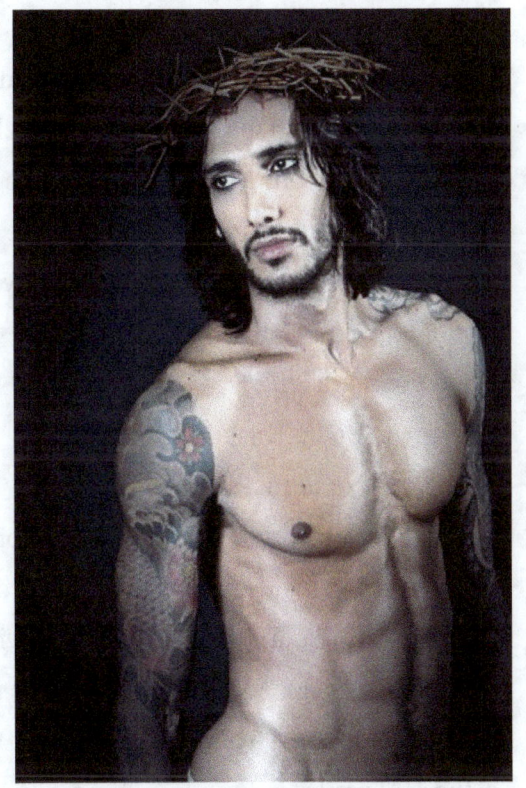

(Brathwaite)

PERFECTION

"I said it wasn't good enough!"

"But Mom, my grades have improved. I'm making a B in math now, why is that not good enough?"

"Cause I'm your mother, and I expect better. I expect an A."

"Did you get an A in math?"

Flames rose in her hazel green eyes. The energy of the room began to stir, signaling the coming storm. "I'm your <u>Mother</u>, *don't* disrespect me!"

"What? I'm just asking. Since you want the A, maybe you should help do the homework."

"You're the one in school. It's your job to get the good grades."

"But, a B is a good grade."

"No to me!" she shrieked.

My mouth opened to respond, but Mother huffed at me and walked out of the room, leaving me alone with the midterm report card with the B in bold ink. I never understood why she was so uptight about math. Not like I was going to use it anytime soon in the 10th grade.

MONSTER BRAIN

I picked up the cordless phone and dialed Dad. He was good at math from his days as a nuclear mechanic in the Navy.

"Dad, I need help on this one problem."

"Ok son, what's the equation?"

"$X-Y=-4+X^2$, with a side of bitch."

"Whoa, what's going on."

"Just mom, being herself again. I showed her the report card and my math grade improved, but it wasn't up to her expectations."

"Ok, so what you gonna do about it?"

"I'll keep studying, but I thought a B is pretty good."

"Well, yeah. It is. Better than the D- you had."

"But everything has to be perfect for her. Perfectly clean, matching close, "A's for grades, and on and on."

Dad sighed on the phone. "It's just her wiring. You learn to work with it and love the woman for who she is. Sometimes it's about keeping quiet and letting her blow out the steam when she's mad about something else."

"Yeah, ok."

"Welcome to *The Taming of the Shrew*...Now, what about that math problem?"

Daniel Cureton

MY BEST GHOST

You know there really wasn't a time that I thought it would come down to the ending of our eight year friendship in which you let go of all that we had built together in favor of isolation, depression, and condescension—it was really a great bother, was it such a great bother, for you to come back and be a good person, like you had been before, instead of succumbing to the influence of cock, heroin filled gingers, and the Norman Bates tones of your inept, suffocating, monster of a mother—no, I guess it was too much since you neither had the spine nor the nerve to stand up and do for yourself except when pressed into a situation into which you had no choice but necessity in order to live, survive, and move forward—and that's all you did, survive—not even that was enough at times it seem; you craved love and companionship, but wished the world would go awry—you waited for me to return from China, looking forward to more adventures, then blamed me for your mother's mouth when I signed a contract for her car—all these things are your problem, bro, buddy oh mine, but only when

MONSTER BRAIN

I was away did you grow up, did you learn to set a boundary; and the first time I set mine with you in the eight years, you laugh, mock, and throw me to the side.

    I thought we were friends; my first true bestie, deepness I had never known: we shared in mutual, and I watched Doctor Who because of you and you grew in your knowledge because of me—we shared dinners, cooking, brunch, and Salt City clubs, you staying in the shadowed corner as I roamed the suds—you helped when no other would, I could trust and depend on you—do you hold my career choice against me? Because I had to move so far away? But I sent postcards, gifts, and love, from Shanghai everyday—I was coming back, to escape that oppressive regime, and the letter with your poem I composed told you that through the slipstream; where did we go wrong, buddy? I can't blame the drugs, but your twisted passivity, and inability to love en mass, paired with hurt from a boy, who played you with needles, and stole the heart you kept in the safe under the sea.

    I thought I knew you Ashton.
    I say goodbye to our friendship:
    June 2010-June 2019

DONATELLO
⚰
(2008–2019)

Mellow kitty,
blackness delight.
We found each other
one fateful night.

New to Salt City,
And Witchy stuff too.
I searched for my soul partner,
a familiar in you.

The shelter called you "Jack."
This was so basic.
I picked up you, Donatello
Joined that day, without nix.

Familiar's Goddess divine,
you loved me as a lover should.
From the first second in my arms,
you saw my knighthood—

MONSTER BRAIN

Rescue for a rescue—two soul creatures.
In a universe wide,
coming together,
no longer to hide.

Ten years we spent
weaving magic of the moon,
divine workings under the sun,
soul filled boon.

You got me thrown out of
not 1, but 2 apartments for breaking pet rules.
But I stuck with you
and found a woman who was so cool.

April took us in,
seeing herself in my plight.
A magical stud with a young kitty
in need of safety's sight.

Long days passed
and short hours
as we lived our lives
and braved the world's sours.

Daniel Cureton

We had comfort—
brothers bond—
as only an animal can
with their human fond.

Then your work was done
and you had to go.
Renal failure came on
so sudden, and slow.

I watched you wither,
waste away, and die.
It broke me inside.
And I knew heartbreak-first time, aye.

What was I to do,
after all those years past.
A decade of my life in Salt City
flew by so fast.

Thank you my dear friend,
we will see each other again,
one day over the rainbow bridge,
in Summerland Fields, amen.

MONSTER BRAIN

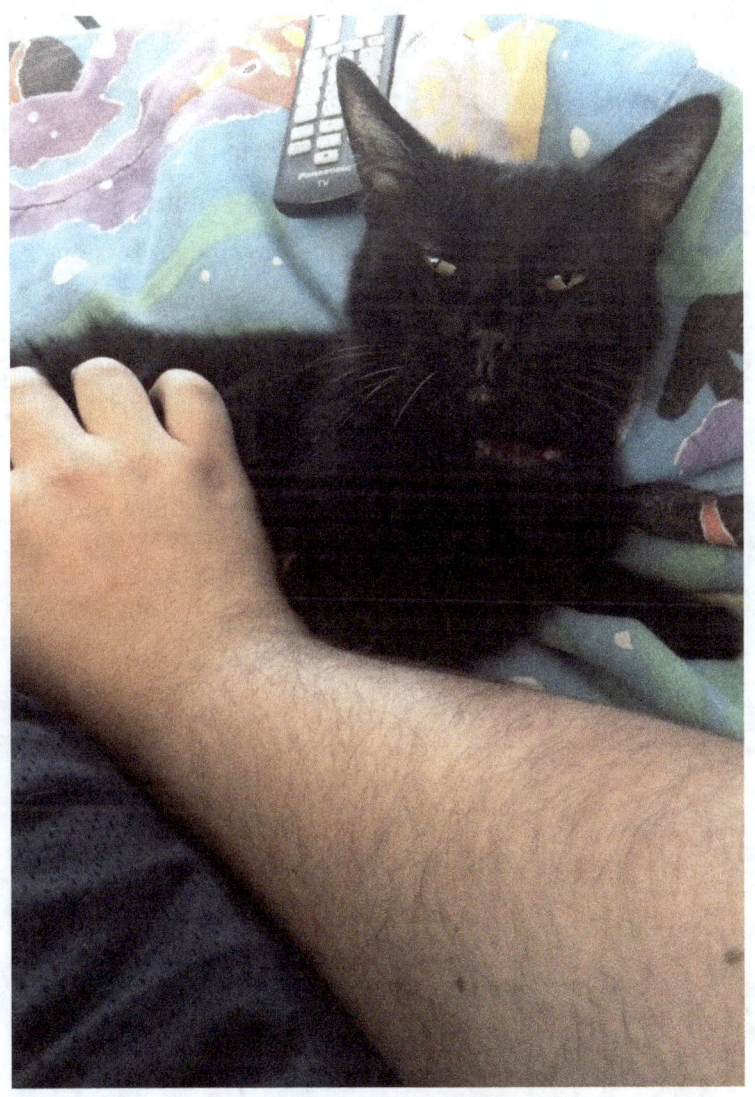

Donatello, July 27, 2016

Daniel Cureton

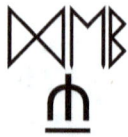

Web, you were the one who gave me a chance, when I came back from China—17 interviews, and you were the one who got me, saw the professional, experienced, and talented professional you wanted to grow the school.

Everything was better when you were there. The days clipped by and I would see you, know you, and feel the community you created. Everything was ok when you were there.

Bonds of friends and collegiality. Strength from the mind, you built us all to heights we didn't know before you entered our lives.

You go suddenly—new job, leaving the bullshit behind—but we are forever changed by your guiding hand and wisdom.

To you, I say thank you, Deb.
My Lagertha.

HEART OF TERROR

It's where it all happened—
in my head—
pick up the knife,
and slice her dead.

Of course, it's embarrassing
to admit you think that way.
But the psyche ward told me
it's not reality, just a stray.

Treatment gave me hope,
to know that "thoughts are thoughts."
And what your brain sends you on OCD
isn't your conscious mind, bought.

You don't desire,
sit and plot,
make sure her backs turned,
and grab the pot.

Daniel Cureton

It's the message of disorder.
Deep inside the fissure it spews,
sends endless waves of terror.
Disconnected, necrotic tissue.

The OCD group:
"You are only responsible for your actions,"
Reassuring a wandering soul in the dark night
that his mind is here, even in sight a fraction.

The knife in the kitchen
is my worst enemy.
Anxiety makes me think I'll grab it
and stab come venally.

Such a fool, the conscious mind,
believing what the terror loop shows.
It doesn't tell us to stay out of the kitchen,
or we'll make a crippling blow.

MONSTER BRAIN

It's not like I pick up the tool,
a cast iron skillet,
and put my weight in—
the Darken hand that wields it.

But the logic of the rational brain,
screams and yells,
"Don't believe it, something is wrong.
it's just a game sent from hell."

Yet, I can't help but feel the fright,
the shame wells inside.
For thinking such thing of my dearest friend,
as soul stands wayside.

Daniel Cureton

ANXIETY'S BANE

You ever felt it:
the uncertainty and distrust?
Your own self a stranger
not knowing who to trust.

Fade in, fade out
the focus is so hard.
Bright lights, enemies—
soul wretched and marred.

The dream quality
slinks across reality,
You are unsure of what's next—
life, dream, or fatality.

Anxiety says to go away,
fold into yourself,
don't go to work,
socialize, or seek help.

MONSTER BRAIN

Everything is out to get you.
Nothing will go right.
You must withdraw from society.
Take immediate flight.

Like the shy cat,
you find yourself imploding
on Anxiety's bane—
foreboding.

Daniel Cureton

FOG

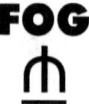

Like the great mists,
you rise.
Infecting the brain waves,
you strive.

Even worse than Red,
you stay.
And surround me
in foggish ways.

I drive home
and you are the road.
I drive back
and you are the road.

I close my eyes—
you invade my mind.
I close my mind—
you invade my eyes.

MONSTER BRAIN

I know the Red Wall,
but you I do not.
Tell me your secret,
so I'm not distraught.

Next I go
and see you there.
I'll know what to do
and not just stare.

You won't scare me,
thinking I've lost it all.
But give me closure,
as I know you're not the white wall.

Daniel Cureton

THE ART OF BREAKING

Nothing is explained and nothing is required. A break is a brake, as they say. No art, but simply the undoing of the mind. The mush of the matter, and the dissolving of the organic floc.

I never expected it to happen to me. I was ok, doing fine, dealing with the stress of life I thought, up until this point. My best friend of 9 years abandoned me after I returned from expat life in Shanghai. My roommate betrayed me, my boss left work, and then the cat died.

It came on me when my long-time companion, a male black cat and my witchy familiar, died after 10 beautiful years together. I never understood pet death could lead to a system shutdown—now I get it—why people take the death of a pet so hard. Donatello was the first one I chose, reared, and saw to the grave. Renal failure—withering condition. And he fought to go, some three hours on my lap, gasping for breath. The loneliness and isolation was terrible, feeling unsafe and unwanted of a city grown into me ten years. But, of other crazy folks it was that:

MONSTER BRAIN

They just say "He was

crazy!

as a

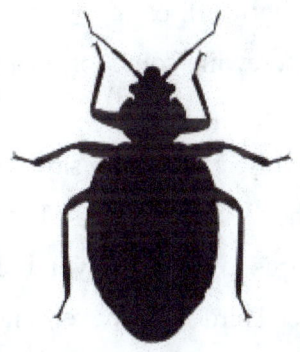

"Lost his damn

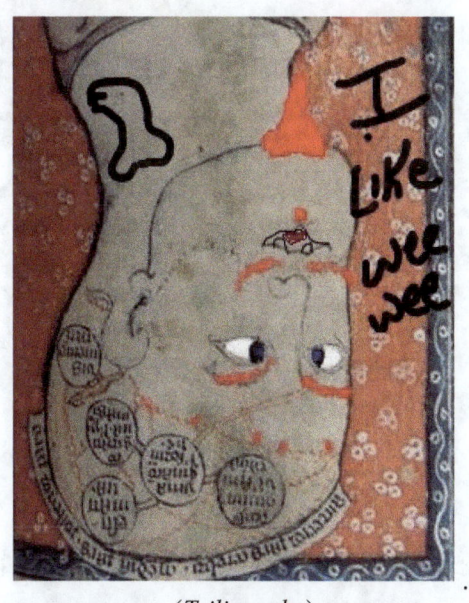

."

(*Trilingual...*)

Daniel Cureton

Well, thankfully I never went crazy, but knowing something of stress, trauma, loss, and hurt can change the very chemistry of your brain.

One day, you're bumbling along fine—handling the stress—: sleeping it off, eating your feelings, working out at the gym, or screwing some lone soul till he prolapses the anus.

It hits suddenly. Those who say "I'm gonna have a break!" But do they? That's stress, but the real break, when your brain turns to farts, and you break wind out the exhaust called the Third eye, never knowing when or where it happens.

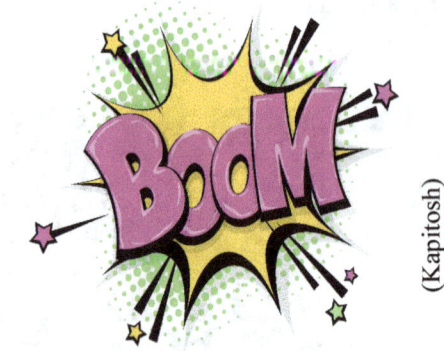

(Kapitosh)

Brain is ~~done~~.

You…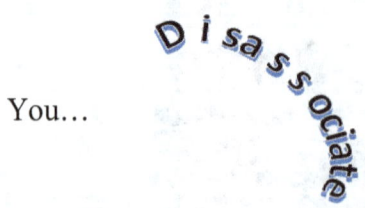

Everything is a

MONSTER BRAIN

Feeling as is your mind has turned to

MUSH

Your rational, scientific

$E=mc^2$ *brainiscertiainyouarejustfeelingtired.*

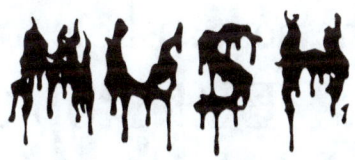

what

happened to all the ? years that I spent honing in my brain, instilling reason and order. It cannot break down!

what is going on here, I can't believe this! I am of sound mind and body—What are these intrusive thoughts??

THEN OCD TURNS ON.

This isn't fair, I should be moving on to the next asshole to screw, or a Ph.D. HEY! Stop that, I don't want to see this horror in my head. Quite talking to me!! SHUT UP!!

MONSTER BRAIN

I WILL not ~~be~~ this person you

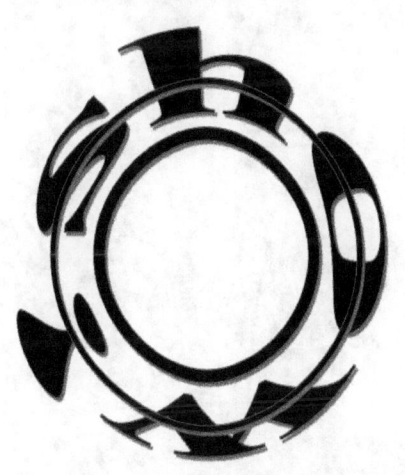

Daniel Cureton

I'd rather

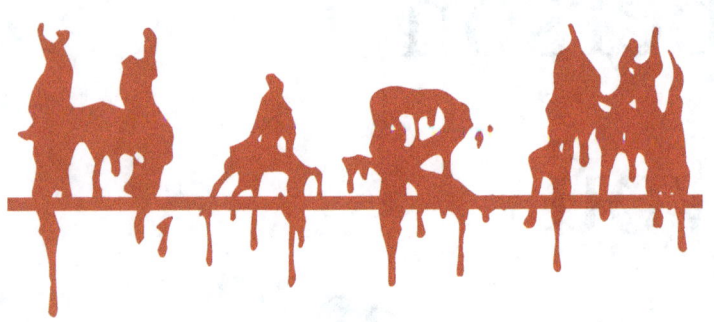

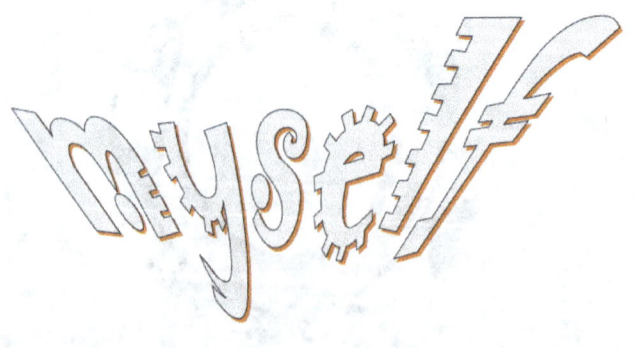

MONSTER BRAIN

THAN someone ELSE

xxx

· · ·

xxx

Daniel Cureton

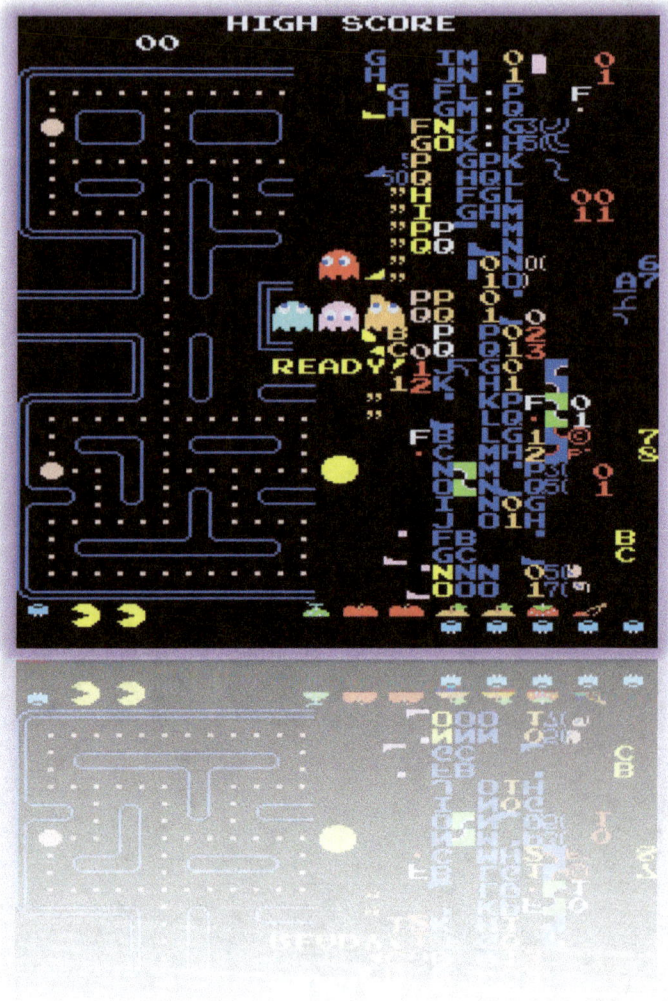

(Killscreen303)

MONSTER BRAIN

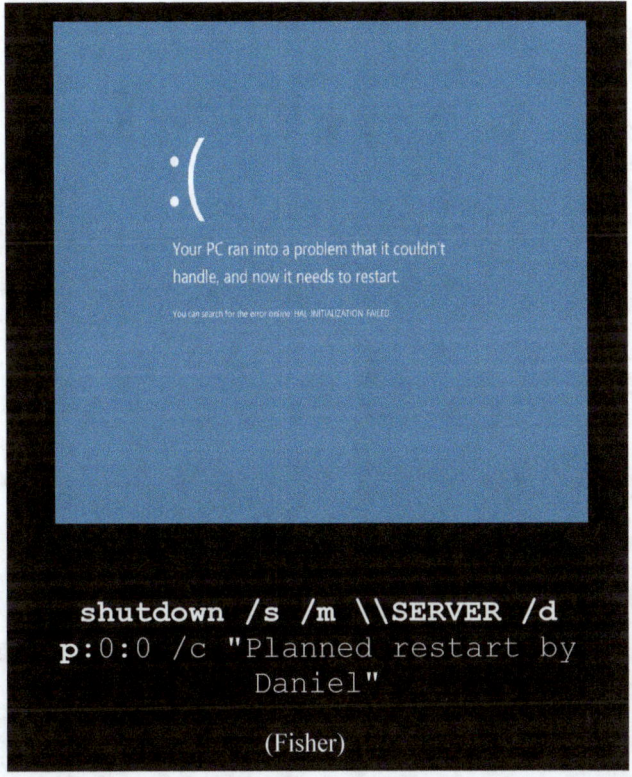

(Fisher)

And so, you break. All the reason and order leaves, and no amount of logic can bring you out of the spiral you went down.

No one says it's ok to feel this way, to feel broken, to see the broken in those moments after the loss.

No one encourages you to seek treatment before it happens, but you know it's the answer.

You call around to get therapy the week you know you're off, but everyone's booked up months ahead, and you feel tossed, let off.

It's all the usual—Ready, Set,

Alone IN A CROWD

A Short Film by OCD

        FLY DOWNARD TOWARD CROWD
EXT. LATE EVENING
BROKEN PERSON is sitting at a table and experiencing the worst of OCD--cartwheels of anxiety. The voices drown out the BROKEN PERSON.

        BROKEN PERSON
    (Looking around at the
    backs of the crowd)
I need help. I don't know what this is I'm feeling. Someone help me.

BROKEN PERSON is also the voice of OCD
        OCD (V.O)
Just kill her. Kill her Now.
        BROKEN PERSON
No! I had plans, have plans. I don't know what's going on. I would rather harm myself than

MONSTER BRAIN

another!!

BROKEN PERSON picks up phone to call a therapist.

   CROWD
  (Collective voice)
Just get over it, you're not really sick. It's all in your head. Just make it go away!

THERAPY VOICEMAIL (V.O)
 (sincere yet unhelpful)
We're sorry, we aren't here right now. The next available appointment is NEVER, so you should just kill yourself.

BROKEN PERSON slams down phone onto ringer, throws hands up.

   BROKEN PERSON
  (Horror Loops being on scream)
Ahhh!!

CUT TO HORROR SCENES

   OCD (V.O)
Yes, 'make me go away.' I'm glad you have no logic to-day Oh! what fun it is to

OCD (V.O. CONT'D)
smash a brain.
Look how easy they strain
So smooth, red, delightful
Nothing more fearful, killing—
and frightful!

CUT TO BROKEN PERSON

BROKEN PERSON is filled with intense panic. Fright appears on their face, they fall to their knees.

BROKEN PERSON
NO...NO

OCD (V.O)
Lade dah, let's try the old plate to the head! Better yet, hammer to the temple instead.

Sharp jolted camera angles zoom onto BROKEN PERSON'S face with angled sunlight illuminating their terror.

OCD (V.O)
Maybe we can hack off the limbs and pretend it's Dicken's little Tims. Or smash in the face, just like the show,

MONSTER BRAIN

and find relief, with the
killing blow.

BROKEN PERSON rocks back and forth in pain.

        OCD (CONT'D)
Better not become like the old
nympha, let out a prayer to
Saint Dymphna!

              CUT TO AERIAL SHOT
CAMERA BLURS FOR INTENSE ANXIETY

        OCD (CONT'D)
You deserve what's your due
For all the hurt, pain, and be-
trayal ensued.

              CUT TO ANGLE DOWNWARD -
           RIGHT SIDE OF BROKEN PERSON
CAMERA GOES MONOCHROME
A bed rolls up into which BROKEN PERSON Crawls.

        BROKEN PERSON
    (Cries in bed)
        CROWD
Why are you crying. Aren't you
strong enough? Face your

Daniel Cureton

CROWD (CONT'D)
fears, and toughen up, scruff!
A typewriter appears on the table beside the bed. BROKEN PERSON gets out of bed turns on the electric typewriter. They sit quietly for a moment, light a cigarette, and start typing

BROKEN PERSON

This last and final note I write
in this dangerous, mental night.
I do not know how to go on,
so I compose this last rhyme long.

What are these thoughts?
Horrible, haunting, distraught
that play on a loop before my eyes
and make me afraid to say goodbye

Nothing helped in fact,
not even the tender loving cat.

The future can't be—for I having cracked
all my dreams, smashed—I now take the whack.

MONSTER BRAIN

ONLY THE ECHOING SOUND OF THE CAR AS HE DROVE INTO THE NIGHT WAS HEARD-- BRAVER THAN THE LONE WANDERER AT DEATH'S DOOR.

Daniel Cureton

INTERMOUNTAIN FAIRIES

The ward was fresh and new—with fear, I tread.
I checked myself and found something of dread.

The mind was wrong with all the terror loops—
I knew it should have been the happy whoops.

The typewriter inked the notes striked by death—
I did not want to take another breath.

The drive to the mystic's magical door
took no time at midnight's slumbering snore.

Gnomes and Goblins, Pixies, and Sylphs—the like
receive me in waiting this frightful night.

Nonesuch creature, quickly pell-mell appeared,
took my willing hand with no-fun sung—drear.

I could not stand the scene inside of me,
what broke did mystify the silver sidhe.

MONSTER BRAIN

Rock and stone do sit—wise to listen long
to stories of bear brain which had gone wrong.

Scribble and scribe, they wait for elder's dye
to get the final seal, and say goodbye.

Sheet of blue did hold the fateful answer—
send the queer—mobile units our prance.

The fairy realm holds the books of shorn wealth
they answer with ease, "better mental health—

"You sought the shaman at E.R.'s longhorn,
Salt Lake Behavioral is not forlorn.

They have a room with a cozy big bed—
give you time to heal anxiety's head.

off you go to another faery realm,
and be of good mind, frame, and body helm."

The week's journey was full of hue of blue;
happiness be found in a new lone crew.

Daniel Cureton

Tears of sadness, turned to tears of relief
as psyche ward eases my anguish and grief.

Locks undone; knobs first turned—closed way no more
seals broken, secrets learned, thoughts washed ashore.

Through altered form—cerebral rendition.
Gateway to better neuro transmission.

THE INTAKE

"I'm afraid," I said as the EMT took my pulse.

"Where will they take me?"

"Salt Lake Behavioral."

"Where is that?"

"7th E," she said. Suddenly the memory of seeing the beige building came back to me memory, the view cattycorner across my work building.

You're kidding. I'm across from work.

The ambulance bumped along. A slow ride to a destiny that scared the hell out of me. I wasn't even as terrified the day I was abandoned in Shanghai. The unknowns—the power—the control…all gone for an eternity, given to the ward.

The arrival was slow. Outside the building the nurses milled about while being unloaded and rolled through double doors. I exited the bed, only in a gown and with the measly white blanket thrown on top of me during the ride.

It felt as if time stretched onwards forever in the waiting room. The homeless man slept in a chair while the young guy prayed loudly to Jesus so Satan wouldn't take his soul. *This* was crazy, not me.

I had to be "inspected..." that's to say, did I have bruises and needle marks, signs to prepare for detox; they rewarded me with some breakfast around 7am.

I wanted to text, to call someone, anyone, but not my mother. What could she do 1700 miles away? Who would be up 7am on a Sunday? The counselor came as I pondered my existentialism for the intake.

"What made you come in this morning?" she asked. "Well, it's not like I really had a choice from the ER." I responded.

"What's going on, that you felt the need to go?"

"I didn't feel right...haven't all week, and I knew something was wrong. I was having crazed images. I've never felt this way, or seen such things I can't turn off, so I knew I had to act."

"I see. And when did this start?"

"After my cat died two weeks ago."

"Aw. Poor kitty, was he old?" she wondered.

"No, 11. He had renal failure. I had him for ten years. I didn't realize it would affect me so much—I thought I was handling it just fine."

"Sometimes things take a while and we don't know it."

"Yeah. So, what's gonna happen to me? I'm new to all this. It must seem pretty pitiful to be in here over my cat."

MONSTER BRAIN

"You'd be surprised as to why people come in—for any reason. We'll get you set up with a bed so you can get some rest, you've been up all night. Just hold on."

The counselor left me to sit, wait, and ponder the rising sun through the window in the east.

DEPRESSION RIOTS

Depression Ward steps off the elevator, shuffling down the labyrinth of doors. Right, forward, left, left again, and ahead—entrance to the Depression Ward.

OCD Man is the first to arrive at the double doors. He takes in the newly posted signs, "High AWOL Risk! WTF."

The group stopped, filled with frayed ends—indistinguishable murmuring is heard as the councilor examines the signs. "I don't know where these would have come from. Which fucker did something?"

The crowd whispered to itself. "Nothing, we were good and sweet and kind. All I do is cry!" laughs the Tooele Woman.

"Could be that David in there finally lost it and tried to kill the nurse for taking his cookie." The group laughs and relaxes into the scene.

"Oh, hey, I think we're on the wrong floor," waves the Son of Odin. "Is this the fourth? We're on the second."

"Ahhhhh!" exclaims everyone as they shuffle back to the elevator. Post-prandial comma was fast

MONSTER BRAIN

acting and weakened the brain reflexes.

"I thought for sure we weren't gonna get out now—'high AWOL!' I wondered why I never saw the Children's Ward across from us till now," shrugged OCD Man.

Taking the journey home, the 2nd floor opened like all the rest: bland, beige, and tight as a virgin twink. The group rolled along, settling back into the chairs and desk, to color or drift into space in the Depression Ward.

Tooele Woman turned to the nurse on duty, "what floor was that with 'high AWOL?'"

"Oh," responds the nurse, "they ain't getting out for a long while. They fight, they run, and can't function without lots of meds and support. Lots of teens."

"Sounds like regular teens to me!" she says, laughing with the nurse.

Tragic Teen leaned over to the OCD Man for chatter, "You know, this has to be the best ward I've been in, and I've been in some awful places around the Wasatch. Y'all are so fun, so happy—I can tell you are all working to get better."

"Yeah, and if they don't let us out, we'll RIOT!" piped in meth granny. "I don' know 'bout you, but 5 days is too long for me."

"Hey, maybe that should be our name" says Tooele Woman.

OCD Man gets a smirk on his face. "Can you imagine it—depression riots—a bunch of depressed corpses rooting for suicide suddenly decide to riot out of the psyche ward? I'm sure half of Salt Lake County would throw us into the next deep hole they find."

"If anything we need a good cheer. So we can practice during the riots!" says Tragic Teen.

"All right then my dear emo,"

WHAT DO WE WANT?
FREEDOM!
WHEN DO WE WANT IT!
MEEeeehhhhh....

sleep

OCD Man looks around. "Well, that ended quickly."

MONSTER BRAIN
A DAY IN THE LIFE OF COMPULSION
⚱

Round 1, 7:00-7:10am, seconds after waking

OCD: Kill them in their sleep.

Daniel: *Love* them in their sleep. *That's what we do.*

OCD: we KILL them in their sleep. *That it's too.*

Daniel: No, we protect— OCD: MURDER them!!

Daniel: NO!! *LOVE,* *krishna is love*

OCD: Too many, not enough time.

Daniel: Too many for what?

OCD: To stab through the heart.

Daniel: WHAT! * krishna is love *

OCD: lade da, just snap his neck!

Daniel: How about we *love* his neck?

OCD: How about we snap it his neck.

Daniel: How about we—OCD: MURDER HIS NECK!

Daniel: SHUT THE FUCK UP!

Daniel Cureton

Round 2, 4-6:23pm.

Daniel: What a wonderful day, I think I—OCD: WILL KILL THE MOTHER FUCKERS, Ahhhahaha!!

Daniel: SHIT!

OCD: You know, it's just a little *slice*. What's the harm?

Daniel *eyeroll*

OCD: Oh Yeah? *Que Various Terror Images*

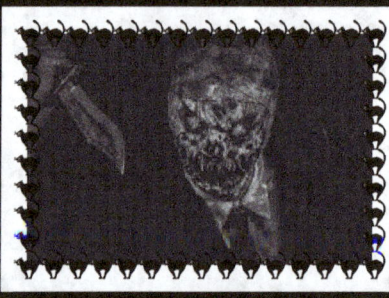

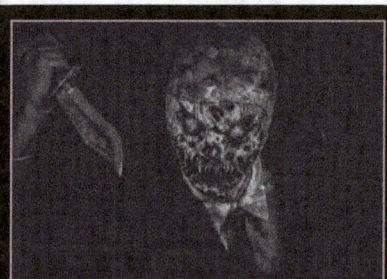

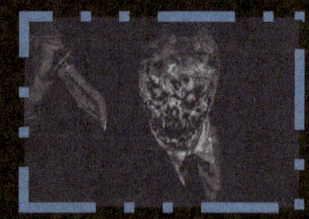

(Max Pixel)

MONSTER BRAIN

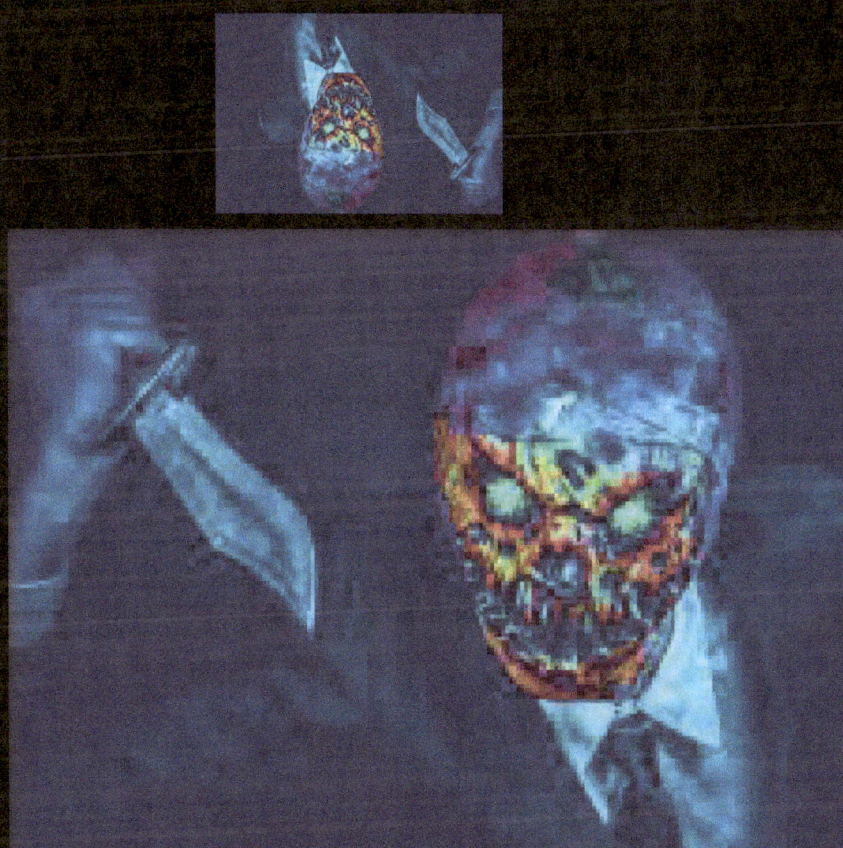

☼♪♫*Krishna Dub* by Mc Yogi♫♪☼

Daniel Cureton

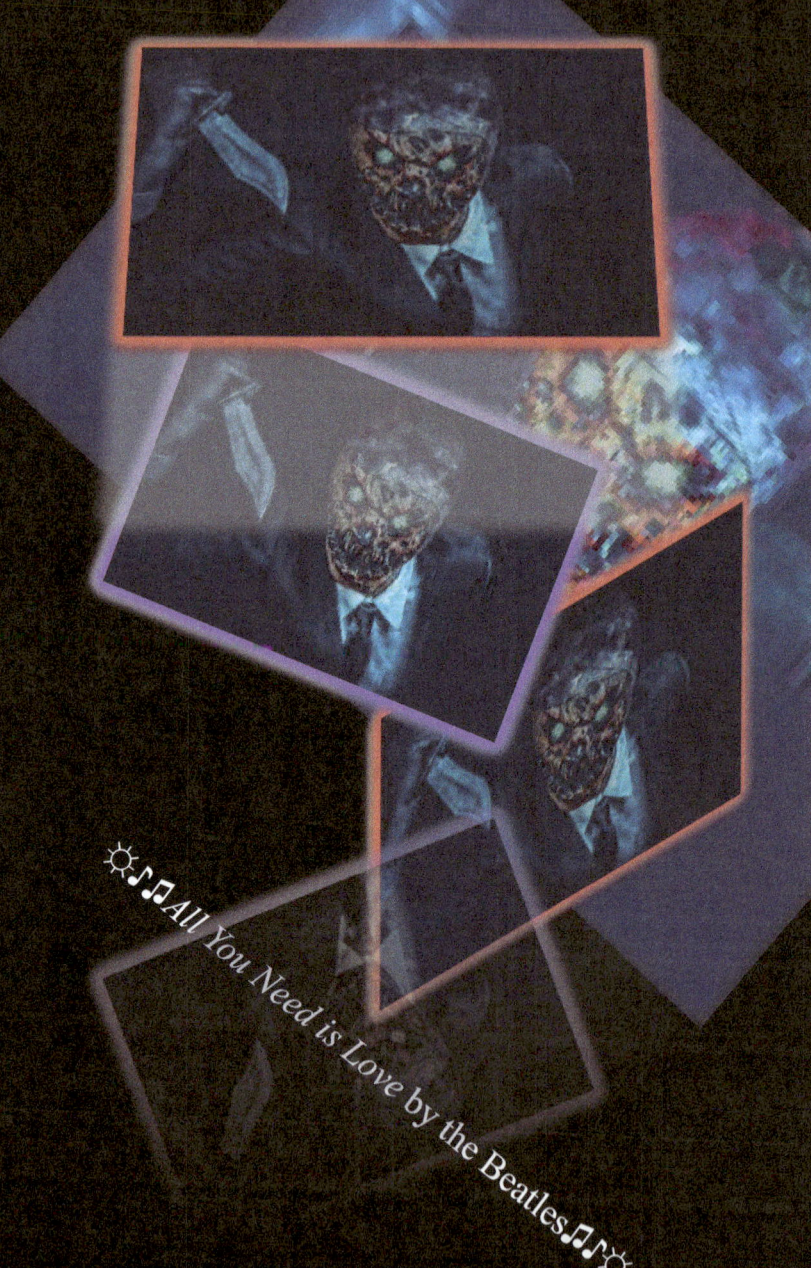

☼♪♫*All You Need is Love by the Beatles*♫♪☼

MONSTER BRAIN

Round 3, 9:01-10:49, before bed

OCD: Murder, murder, murder, everywhere—murder is good!

OCD: No, murder is not ~~good~~, it is bad!

Daniel: No, murder is ~~good~~!

OCD: murder is ~~good~~! OCD/Daniel: Murder is ~~so good~~!

Daniel: ~~murder is good~~!

OCD: murder is-Daniel: bad-OCD: heavenly!

Daniel: No, it is unethical!

77

Daniel Cureton

Daniel: NO, STOP TWISTING MY WORDS!

OCD: Kill them all, big and small, kill them all!

Daniel: ~~Kill~~ LOVE them all, big and small, ~~kill~~ LOVE them all!

MONSTER BRAIN

NAOMI: 1 ○ OCD: 0

Dear Naomi,

How do I say thanks to you for what you have done, in saving me from myself?

The psychiatrist didn't take interest, just thought I was depressed. You though…you knew, you suspected. I am eternally grateful for the experienced, and confident professionals who take their craft as seriously as you. Your intuition, your meetings, and your knowledge said, "Hey, I bet this guy has OCD."

Naomi: 1 - **OCD**: 0

Yes! The day you handed me the article allowed me to return to my body. I felt the joy of understanding their was hope. I felt the excitement in understanding I wasn't a criminal, desiring things that were at complete odds with my core being. I wasn't going to jail, or going to be institutionalized. I simply had a brain disorder.

To you, Naomi, thank you for following your hunch, for being interested, for caring, and showing me the way to recovery.

Forever in Your Debt

Daniel Cureton

PURE O

Harm is born within humans,
something about primal lust,
and the poet's pen turns
red guts to dust.

Something about primal lust,
as Pure O, Harm OCD it is known.
Red guts to dust
that the film loop has shown.

As Pure O, Harm OCD it is known,
shows me all the ways to hurt.
That the film loop has shown,
I feel like fucking dirt.

Show me all the ways to hurt.
My mind is terrible.
I feel like fucking dirt.
Suicide is the only thing bearable.

MONSTER BRAIN

My mind is terrible,
I'm going mad.
Suicide is the only thing bearable,
offing myself is better.

I'm going mad,
I am not this horrible human.
Offing myself is better—
I want to be the Goddess' lumen.

Daniel Cureton

THE POSE

The chaos of the real world
left behind the door
as we stretch into a pose.

Shiva Nataraja dance,
on the floor we roll
doing the divine lingam.

Up, down, around, and back through.
Awaken the snake
lying at the base of the spine.

The mind forgets what's within,
releasing the pressure
of the broken spirit's bane.

Yoga's third eye opens now—
sight for the future,
vision for destiny bold.

MONSTER BRAIN

WESTERN UNION TELEGRAM

W. P. MARSHALL, CHAIRMAN OF THE BOARD
R. W. McFALL, PRESIDENT

NO. WDS-CL. OF SVC	PD. OR COLL.	CASH. NO.	CHARGE TO THE ACCOUNT OF	TIME FILED
132	CALL	.75¢	Daniel Cureton, poet	12:21 Pm

To. The Man at the Counter Who Served Lunch

Street and No. 3802 S 700 E, Salt Lake City, UT 84106

Care of or Apt. No. _____ Destination Cafeteria 20 19 AD

Your smile was a bridge to the Summerlands, taking me away to a place I longed to go.

Ever friendly, the sincerity in your question "How are you today?" could be felt as deeply as the blackness of the night sky.

You beamed with the energy of the stars, traversing the ravine to lift me out of the pit into which I had fallen.

Thank you for allowing me to exist in the moments with you as I was, as you served up a meal.

With the generosity of a most kind soul, you are content in the happiness of service. Filled with the Christ charity, the patience of Quan Yin, and empathy for the humans who were lost.

Daniel Cureton

THE RED WALL

Giant, throbbing barrier.
It came as I drove home one night—
a buttering, brooding,
blistering sight.

I had no idea what I was seeing
except the mountains were gone.
Where were the Wasatch,
sturdy, tall, and strong?

Fleshy, froth—froopy.
Drippy, demon—droopy.
Quivering, quaking—quickening.
Sliming, slithering—sickening.

You intruded into my mind,
blocked neurons from view.
How do I look past what's inside
without bidding myself adieu?

MONSTER BRAIN

Moment of the break,
I thought you were "The Blessing,"
but Jack was a fantasy
and you were just all me stressing.

Inconceivable, incoherent—incongruity,
impose, implant—impurity
Dispose, destruction—disuse,
devour, discerption—detinue.

Such pain, loneliness never before known.
Friendships broken, bonds distrusted
I didn't know my life had become so—
mental health, critique, universal must.

Much like Torchwood's immortality,
I feared to come apart
Were you trying to protect my consciousness—
wall of red, bleeding heart?

Daniel Cureton

Oh Brenda, there is no shame in crying. You are lost on the ship of souls, here in the ward. Through the tears, flowing as streams into the emotion Nile; you banish all the fears. Let it go, all out, with the bad and good, and look at life for what is worthy of your embrace. Love lost, but new friends found—we are comrades in the war of the mind; and you and I rejoice together as soulmates. Come hither, dear Brenda, and be one with me as we sail the depression sea.

MONSTER BRAIN

MY NURSES

☼ The Morning Shift ☼

You were there, to greet me, with the witchy ways—sister of the craft. You saw the same kindred. You gave the message from Cam, "rawr," which tickled you pink to read the intimates of two souls. Having been where I had been, you knew I would be ok. You were kind to me when I was most vulnerable. To you, I thank you for easing my anguish and uplifting me to the ledge to grab hold to.

◯ The Day Shift ◯

You made life good. Thanks for all the naps. You knew I was so tired, brain tired, dead tired. The meds made it worse, and I was trying my best but couldn't stay up in the chair. The couch was hard, and the noise from the TV harder. The laughter you encouraged eased our pain, and made life chill from all the stress of the world.

✧ The Night Shift ✧

Thank you for how attentive to your duties you were. You checked every 15 minutes, waking us up to see if we were dead—yet you kept us alive. As we fell asleep each day, you made sure at least that we were worn down and ready for the counseling, the therapy, yoga, and 3 square meals so we would sleep at night. I won't miss the ruffle of sheets, the flash light in my face, or the movement of feet. But thanks, thanks for watching out.

Daniel Cureton

TO HAVE A CAM

The night was young and free,
fueled by the coffee and bean;
lending the energy of tomorrow
with potential, thought, and desire.

Sweet scent of the eye,
Peeling the layers off.
Clothes falling away,
in the mind's world.

The first touch came
like a warmth through the skin—
two halves become whole sucking
through the self-wind.

The universe before us,
Cam on the scene,
giving radiance to beam
and beauty to shape.

MONSTER BRAIN

Understanding where there is none.
Others block the way,
you lay the path
knowing what can be done.

Manifest creature of dreams,
spilling secrets of shadow—
ecstasy untouched—
beating, one being.

Daniel Cureton

WHITE PILL

A Short Film

INT. MEDICAL OFFICE—EARLY MORNING
DOCTOR walks in. Camera is blurred at angle from table to only see DOCTOR's body. His face is never seen.

>DOCTOR
>
>Hello Mr....OCD, how are we feeling today?
>
>MR. OCD
>
>(Deadpan face)
>
>Like my guts are being torn up. And yourself?
>
>DOCTOR
>
>Yes, all fine. You're here 'cause you were at the psyche ward and need med management? We can do that. They have you on Prozac?

MONSTER BRAIN

        MR. OCD (V.O)

Hospital said it was Prozac. Don't want those—gives me leg spasms

    (Voiced)

Ah, Prozac, and some other that makes me sleep… Cymbal?

MR. OCD shakes head while looking at the floor trying to shake off confusion. DOCTOR sits down in chair across from MR. OCD.
CAMERA SHOWS DOCTOR'S TORSO WITH LEGS CROSSED.

        DOCTOR (O.S)

Prozac. Well, you don't need it, and the leg spasm concern me. We'll switch you to Lexapro and go from there—see how you are in a month.

CAMERA CLOSE UP ON MR. OCD.

        MR. OCD (V.O)

Onward to Lexapro. *Sigh* That works! How long?

Uncertain panic starts to hit MR. OCD.

DOCTOR (O.S)
Generally, we like a trial for a month-

MR. OCD slowly closes his eyes.
CAMERA ON LIPS.

MR. OCD (O.S)
(while DOCTOR talks)
Uh huh.

Intense wave of unfocused anxiety hits MR. OCD.
LIGHT AND HEAT INTENSITY INCREASE IN ROOM.
Sound becomes more muffled as DOCTOR speaks.

DOCTOR (CONT'D)
-see how you do. Is that ok for you?
(Pause)
Mr. OCD, are you alright?

MR. OCD
Yes, doctor, just feel terrible inside. I'm being eaten alive it seems.

SOUND IS SUDDENLY SHARP AND PIERCING.

MONSTER BRAIN

Door closes in medical office, jolting MR. OCD, who quickly turns to look. CAMERA CLOSE UP ON LEFT SIDE OF FACE FOR MR. OCD'S TURN.
Car honks outside. After standing, MR. OCD resists the urge to run to the window.

        DOCTOR

   Those who want to get better, do. You're here, so keep going.

MR. OCD Glares in DOCTOR'S direction. He is experiencing rapid mood swings. CAMERA SHAKES SLIGHTLY.

        MR. OCD (V.O)
   (Angrily)
   Bastard, I know that! I have shit to do before this bitch gets me.

   (Voiced with effort)
   One day at a time, better than another minute this way.

DOCTOR turns to his computer screen. Continues in medical jargon.

DOCTOR (CONT'D)
You'll need to give it a few weeks to build up, but the SSRI will help inhibit the selective serafeelin reuptake frazlemore—Serotonix—frrresss...

CAMERA ON TORSO OF MR. OCD AS BREATHING INTENSIFIES.

DOCTOR (CONT'D)
(long, drawn out, and sultry.)

DOCTOR (CONT'D)
you'll *feeeeeeel* better.

MR. OCD tries not to cry but shows tears. Confused, MR. OCD is trying not to hyperventilate

MR. OCD
(Breathy)
Ok. I guess, 10mg isn't, so bad.

DOCTOR (V.O.)
Patient willing, will try new meds. Reevaluate in 30 days. Include therapy options.

MONSTER BRAIN

MR. OCD exits. DOCTOR types notes.
WHITE PILL IS SEEN ON TABLE WITH DOCTOR BLURRED IN BACKGROUND.

           FADE OUT

Daniel Cureton

NOTE TO SELF

It's ok to feel bad. To feel the sense of dread.
You are new to this, and don't know how it's fed.
You broke inside, and formed something new.
How you handle, how you chose, is now up to you.

Take strength in family, friends, and kindreds.
The ancestors watch over.

Be kind to yourself, life can be lived again.
You have so much to do, and live for.

Don't give up now. Pass the test, and come out better
from the universes' forge than when you went in.

Shining blade, purity in heart, and determined mind.
You will succeed, and find the finish line!

MONSTER BRAIN

WHAT ISN'T RIGHT: A CATALOGUE

It just doesn't sit right with me, I feel compelled to do it again. I am stuck in the loop of my mind. My body hurts—my muscles ache—my teeth clatter, with the catalogue of items, that aren't correct, till I do it again, again, and AGAIN:

- Facing the same direction a vehicle is moving.
- Pulling my hair out of my leg below the knee.
- Grinding these two teeth together till they line up perfectly.
- Walking on one side of the side walk.
- Sniffing the smell of new money, newsprint, books, and magazines.
- Tapping the pen on my teeth.
- Holding my breath till I get that rush, especially as I pass through a yellow light while driving.
- The way the books line up on the shelf.
- The straight line my canned food is supposed to make.
- The number of times I sniff the scent of pits.

Daniel Cureton

- Waiting too long to drink after I swallowed the delicious food.
- Rewinding the movie since I know I missed a word in the subtitles.
- TASCHEN art books which print paintings on two pages, but not fully, so only 1/3 of the painting is on one page and the other 2/3 on the other, creating a seam that is ungodly in the image due to the spine of the book.
- How many times I pet the dog or cat.
- Ending my counting on a prime number.
- Lathering up the soap on my hands.
- The position in which I awake after sleeping.
- Turning my head to look at my friend.
- The color order of the pens on my desk.
- The loops I need to make around the grocery store before I buy tomatoes.
- Sitting at the same desk all semester in college.
- How many times I stroke my cock before I cum.
- Avoiding the cracks on the pavement.
- Passing the mirror with my arm over my head and looking upwards.
- Rereading the paragraph to make sure I didn't miss a word.
- Counting the change in my pocket.
- Listening to the same song without end in my mind,

MONSTER BRAIN

on the radio, or my computer.
- The intensity with which I puff air through my nose.
- Clenching my butt cheeks as I walk.
- Checking the stove to make sure I didn't accidently put the baby or cat inside.
- The number of times and intensity by which I blink.
- The arrangement of the knives in the kitchen.
- The placement of people around the dinner table in the order I did not choose for them.
- Counting the cracks in the side walk before I reach school.
- The number of tiles on the ceiling.
- A stanza being split between two pages.
- Staying a certain feet away from people.
- The number of hairs on my head/their length.
- How many chews I do before I swallow my food.
- Drinking my drink from the same side of the glass.
- Sitting on the far or near side of the table at a restaurant, depending on if I was first or second in line as we sat down at the table being seated by the host.
- And everything else that just. *Isn't.* **RIGHT!**

Daniel Cureton

THE BLUR

It comes from the lights
and the sounds hung in the air.
The blaze of the phone
ringing its dare.

No one remembers,
till they strike their recall
and text, email, message,
admitting they dropped the ball.

Anxiety says you can't focus.
The pressure on the forehead
overwhelms you while you sit
wishing you were dead.

Nothing helps.
Only sleep,
where you dream the problems
with no dip in the beat.

MONSTER BRAIN

Pills, meds, rest.
What else can be done?
Break from social media,
but you haven't won.

It comes and goes,
forever present and waiting.
The blur in reality
with no escaping.

FATIGUE

1.
I lie in bed with time ticking
I should rise, but fatigue's pricking
So, I continue
Like some detinue
can't bear the smile, mimicking.

2.
Never had I known it was this
all those years in Aries bliss
Not knowing, ok
Not feeling, ok
What will it take to feel again?

3.
Email pings, low sound with a sting
What message today will it bring
never to rise again
soul's tender lutein
hours speed by, work a miss.

MONSTER BRAIN

4.

I open the phone looking around
Cute bodies and flesh to be found
A druther to go through
No desire imbued
To depression's will I am bound.

Daniel Cureton

OCD CENTER

Hope comes north
on high hills seen.
From valley of salt,
and pioneer's bean.

OCD and Anxiety Center—
Bountiful bond.
Never told its secret
till its way I was bound,

Heading north, on I-15
The 20-mile drive was a breeze.
Slow and steady, round the course
the mountain rumbled, and sneezed.

Such a place,
a bastion of hope,
lighting the way
for each broken bloke.

MONSTER BRAIN

Knowledge—

powerful tight rope tether.

We found community,

and put the pieces back together.

Daniel Cureton

TO AARON

You didn't rock a pencil stache
but a cool chic.
You were a dappered dash
and not a speak easy sneak.

Roll camera, set, action
we came to be friends.
Queer library, bearaction,
you were a twinky then.

You almost came to China
I said wait, I'll be home.
You set me up with reels
on the endless loop's roam.

I wasn't sure till I left
that I'd make the movies.
Film, shootem' and roll, boy
and don't work at Brewvies.

MONSTER BRAIN

You were there when things went bad—
Depressions' knowledge your key.
Such dripping WASP support,
a two-bit monstrosity.

Thanks, deaf friend,
for telling me about the artist colony.
How to move up in the world,
bleeding Ektachrome dies of Volany.

No more blood's bane due,
—slitting wrists, hollowed and dry,
In the car I saw the real Aaron,
not the shelled out schlock of a guy.

Daniel Cureton

DIRTY DIAPER

The damned child poops all day long
What am I to do?
If I touch the poo,
I know I will die blue.

What am I to do?
The germs are deadly.
I know I will die blue
from contamination steadily

The germs are deadly.
Haven't you read WebMD?
From contamination steadily,
the only thing will be sickness, death, and entropy.

Haven't you read WebMD?
There are thousands of pages to feed your anxiety.
The only thing will be sickness, death, and entropy
if you don't take care to protect yourself wildly.

MONSTER BRAIN

The are thousands of pages to feed your anxiety.
No one tells you not to throw the baby out with the diaper
If you don't take care to protect yourself wildly,
a droplet may spill on your skin like a viper.

No one tells you not to throw the baby out with the diaper.
You should have never had kids in the first place.
A droplet may spill on your skin like a viper.
You will sizzle and die—

What a waste.

Five Nights at Darby's

For when the anxiety hit, only one I could turn to was found.

I didn't know she knew me so deeply—

Verily, to you *моя дорогая подруга,* I was bound—

Ever watching me from shadow's keeply.

MONSTER BRAIN

New feelings ire,

Inside the strong queer.

Gone is confidence's crown,

Honed in from memory's brawn,

Tempered with life's obsolescence,

Set down as law in the organic machine.

Angst's putrid center,

Thwarting growth on future's credit, splinters.

Daniel Cureton

Darby comes to the scene,

Arms wide, open.

Refuse with space unseen.

Bed and key, Goddess token.

Yearning—san lien—only for companion's delight.
'

Soul and sister—*товарищ*, shining knight.

MONSTER BRAIN

BRAIN TRIPPIN'

"I said oh well!! Don't care." he said nonchalant as the anxiety welled inside. The mental struggle was exhausting, the unrelenting grind of obsessive compulsive disorder never relented on the organic machine.

"Well Daniel, how about try this fry pan on for size. See how hard it hits the brain with ease?" said OCD

"I don't care. I don't want to care about fry pan weights on skulls."

"Now, let's try to see the exploding brains that fly out when you strike."

"Ugh, disgusting. Too bad it's a watermelon now."

"Problem solved" smiled OCD. "We'll just reset the loop."

Daniel sat in the chair, rubbing his temple. The exhausting from the compulsion was tiring, even just a few hours into the work day. He stood up to get some fresh air, but OCD threw another scene at him before he could make it outside.

"How about the body being chopped on the

counter. Don't you enjoy the slow slice of flesh, just like *Saw*?"

"Shut up!" Daniel let out a sigh as he entered the elevator. A ping of fear struck through the anxiety, guilt at such twisted images playing out on loop.

A friend, Jazzy, saw Daniel in the hallway making his exit to the car garage, "Hey stud, where are you going."

"Oh, to clear my mind."

"Yeah? How you feeling, it's only been two weeks since you got back."

"Some days better than others. It's hard with still sorting out which meds are gonna work. They put me on Lexapro, so we'll see."

"Awesome!" said Jazzy with a wink. "Hey, want to get lunch? I want to talk about lover boy in IT. Ugh! I don't know, somedays I want to jump his bones, but then my boss walks by and I want to jump his too!"

"Why not have both? You could do a spit roast," offered Daniel with a sly grin.

Jazzy gave him a blank look, "What's that."

"Oh, honey. I need to fill you in over a good, fat, polish sausage from J. Dawgs!"

STUDIO OF APOLLO

The ropes slams
and the weights are high.
I step onto the scale
and have nothing to deny.

You were there, when few others were
steady, helpful,
Fitness Together;
not the blur—not the doubtful.

All the trainers
ever present and reliable.
One team united,
brothered, untrifled,

To you,
I have to thank
for being with me
and filling my tank:

Daniel Cureton

Jacob—not juvy jones.
The Man
"Cureton not the Puritan—Steady Eddy."
6'8 stud of pure delight
kindness, friendship,
and genuine sincerity.

Desi,
kindred betch soul,
blunt for days.
Never trusting I'm pushing hard
or hard enough for her.

Drew,
figuring out fatherhood.
How we talked literature
and comics to get you ready for grad school.

Militant Alison,
crazy moves and motions
not thinking that your notions
were fit for this bear—
100 lbs. too heavy.

MONSTER BRAIN

Health and wellness
saving me from myself—
the decade of poverty
and decline into my 30s.

Apollo himself proud
for the progress made.
More to go, but you keep me on track
even when my mind bails and wades.

I knew what had to be done.
You knew what could be achieved.
I provide the will,
the studio provides belief.

Daniel Cureton

THE LONG, LONG SHOWER

If I turn the knob as so, no germs will flow
nothing but clean, purified, tap water will blow.

Last time I was here for only two hours,
but this time I know I can make it dour.

To get our of here in 20 minutes is the dream.
But it's so far off, much further than this stream.

Why can't I be like him, the hubby
and get my ass out in 30 minutes from this tubby.

The germs plague my mind and body,
but is it worth the hours lost next to the potty.

I'm as clean can I get, soaping up my hands
if I rub all over quickly, and wash down as planned.

My legs get tired, and my skin is prune.
I need a chair in here, to get through this boon.

MONSTER BRAIN

I thought I'd run out of hot water by now—
three hours flew by, but how?

I was so intent on getting clean
I didn't see time tick by unseen.

No one else understands my plight,
that germs will kill me tonight.

No music helps, or thoughts of being dry.
Why must I suffer so, helpless, in the shower's eye?

What I am to do, stuck in my obsession?
I am a prisoner in this title oppression.

Daniel Cureton

HYPOCHONDRIASIS

Dear World,

    Here I die. I write my note of my last breath of life. The cough came suddenly, the pounding headache too. Something unexpected; more than the last time—too soon.

    I give you the complete list of causes, that I have known for years, would be my executioner:

    The germs, from the door know, those must be the cause. The toilet seat in the locker room, that filth did me in.

    The person who sneezed on the bus, it had to be their disease.

    The tumor, I always suspected, exploding in my head.

    I handled my cousin's rat—the boil is the plague—the scratch it gave me is Lockjaw—shutting tight my trap.

    No compress or herbs can heal a bruise. The fall I took caused internal bleeding. Any hour the color will drain away leaving me the cold shell of person.

    As always, it's cancer—must be the quick

MONSTER BRAIN

kind that doesn't take its time.

Either way, a few days and I'm done. I leave you everything, no need to repugn. Share my memory. This new life, will be sickness free.

Till next we meet.

Daniel Cureton

LET THE BODIES HIT THE ROAD

The bump in the road was a body.
I know it.
I must turn around.
If I don't check the streets this time,
a mangled corpse will be found.

I drove 10 miles under,
speed limit 30.
The impact sent me high
as I rode over the child
and the police passed by.

What was I to do??
Go back and check,
turn around and flip a U
to see If the body was a wreck!

Oh, the anguish of the thought
that I had hit Babushka,
"May I see the Manager" Karen,

MONSTER BRAIN

or Timmy the homeless guy
who should not meet Charon.

Brakes wearing through,
driving around this cirque,
where was the proof in my mind?
Evidence I needed strewn about
to confirm I wasn't kind.

As the speedometer defied me,
I never made it to work.
The guilt welled inside,
this feeling I couldn't shirk.

Minutes flew by
to portent surprise—
morpus empty in the wend
I arrived to see a pothole,
not my expired friend.

No one could love such a creature.
Black bag of shame.
All they see is machine,
obsession of the key
and powerless Dramamine.

Daniel Cureton

One day I may stop,
as the octagon sign suggest
It's much harder than it looks—
starving the monster—
that hides in every nook.

I drive on through,
keep on going, blue.
Feeling such a load
let the bodies hit the road.

THE SKIN PICKER

The flesh rolls back.
Blood flows free,
the pain opens the crack—
Compulsion silences its plea.

Blood flows free,
as the obsession takes—
Compulsion silences its plea
as the finger nail scrapes.

As the obsession takes
the dermatillomania soul aghast—
as the finger nail makes
the chagrined face downcast.

the dermatillomania soul aghast,
hands the tool of pain.
The chagrined face downcast,
Anxiety's struggle, OCD brain.

HETEROFLEXIBLE?

You could suck off every jock in this locker room and swallow their loads like horchata!

startle "WTF!?"

Every dick I suck means I'm gayer than the rest.

"What, I don't suck dick!"

Yeah bro, it's the hottest thing.

"OMG, what are you talking about."

Why don't you try it, you might like it enough to switch.

"Um, seeing that I don't get a twitch even for guys, I think I'm ok."

Just look at how the light hits his eyes.

"Ugh, I hate this."

Those sculpted muscles and throbbing quads... yum!

"I want to seriously barf."

What, so gay is wrong?

"No, but I have no attraction to dudes, yet you keep saying it over and over, nonstop, any dude I look at!"

Have you tried it?

"No, why do I need to? I get rock hard for pussy.

MONSTER BRAIN

Case closed"

But, what if...

Sigh "Homosexual-OCD"

How about that hot interracial gay Asian bareback cum pie porno you saw pop up other night on Pornhub. You know that Thai twink getting slammed by that Mexican muscle bear was delicious. *Shows pop-up ad*

"Now this is really making me upset. But you know what, I'm not bothered. Love is love. Gay, straight, bi, trans, cis, queer, all sex is good. I know who am I. Show away dude!"

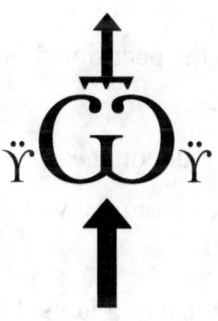

Daniel Cureton

DEBUSSY'S IDYLL

To escape the mind flayer
that comes in the night—
in the day,
in the hour, and
the minute—
music is needed.

The flayer feasts—the occasional insanity is good
for mental health—
but, there is a peaceful cottage
in the cogs, far away from the world.

After the long languish of a lapped lunatical day—
the sense and scene percipient before me—
Hue of Blue and *White Pill*, keep me twined
before I fall into the void, blind.

Anxiety fades
replaced by the serene beauty of the perfect place.
Forests filled with the hums of song birds,
scent of meadow mountains flowers perfume

MONSTER BRAIN

as I nap under the shade of an oaken tree.
Much like *Walden*,
we sit and slumber,
feel firm ground under
and find renewal in the passages of days without humans.

Debussy sounds a round.
The ivories of the relaxing sound—
such pleasant beauty, as light shines in the canopy
and measures out existence in plangent pings—

Music brings ease.
Fortifying,
threads that make up existence
called the universe's art:

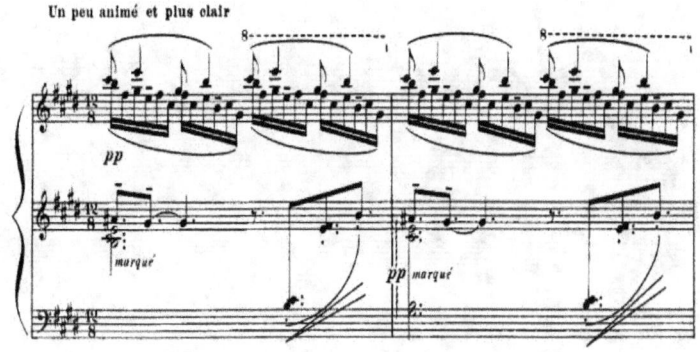

(Debussy, Excerpt 1 from Images I L105 & Images II
L105, No. 4 Cloches à travers les feuilles)

Daniel Cureton

Hammer strikes wound ding
killing blows to anxiety's wing—
OCD exhausts its ring—
Under the piano's succulent string.

Debussy, Beethoven, Mozart
focusing mind for a minute,
fill the neurons—
stop gaps in organic cracks—

Tranquil peace in the notes rung
through ears buzzing, sung.

Claude, you show the way.
Complex rhymes take
my troubled soul away.

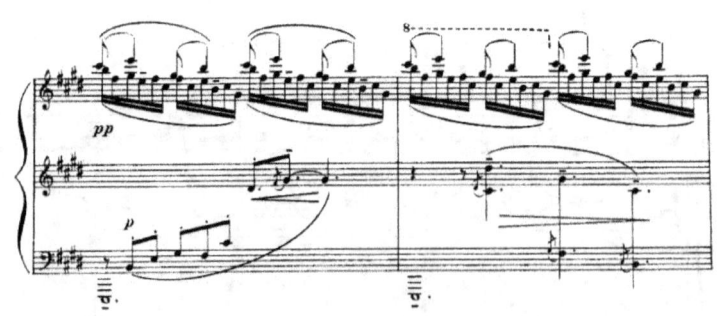

(Debussy, Excerpt 2 from Images I L105 & Images II L105,
No. 4 Cloches à travers les feuilles)

MONSTER BRAIN

Waiting for the noise to die,
under the stroke of felt—
worth measures in gold—scores
pastoral beauty, the counter point
bringing me home.

The breezed air sweeps away the world of tomorrow
enchantment and puerility.
The heartbeat of the harmony as I sleep peacefully
stress vanquished, wanderer lost no more.

but found, layers of flowing rind
I enter my world—Idyll of the Mind.

Daniel Cureton

TRICHOTILLOMANIA

Every pull felt right
satisfaction guaranteed to last.
Seconds, before I wanted—needed another.

"Oh!" the brain says. "Yes, keep pulling
Till there is no more!"
Again, again, again—"that neck's gonna hurt!"

The tug begins
and the hair uncurls,
as I slip my finger, between the furl.

Feel the pressure
of the root yank out
and the rupture of flesh, lout.

"Say it again, say it with me," mind says
"All those hairs, don't look right.
Be sure to use all your strength and might."

MONSTER BRAIN

You know you want to, it's who you are—
resistance is futile, Locutus would say,
do the compulsion, only this way.

Grab the tweezers,
use your nail
it does matter how it's done.

"The only thing I require is your time."
The hours of your life willed away
in obedience to your trichotillomania obsession.

Daniel Cureton

THAT DAMNED LOCK

I feel sick inside when I have to check that lock.
I know what's happened, I very much comprehend
the compulsion of this organic rock.

It's too bad the mechanism isn't a shlock.
If it breaks, I'd rather not go to mend.
I feel sick inside, when I have to check the lock.

I wish there was a clock
to turn the hand of time to wend,
the compulsion of this organic rock.

I wish I knew if I'm the only one on the block
who deals with the checking tend.
I feel sick inside, when I have to check that lock.

If anyone knew, then I know they would mock
I don't want to be awkward, or offend—
the compulsion of this organic rock.
Life will never be the same cause of compulsion's shock.

MONSTER BRAIN

I'll be alone forever—
shamed to show a friend
I feel sick inside, when I have to check the lock—
the compulsion of this organic rock.

Daniel Cureton

LOVE THE CHILDREN

An angel's flesh
so supple, so new,
flash before the school bus
in the tight jean hue.

I cannot—I will not be OCD brain,
you fucking liar.
My hands cover face
and my thoughts become ire.

I know I am not the monster inside
that tells me children as desire.
It's the intrusive thoughts of a sickened head—
Anxiety's lies, in the pedophile's mire.

Sexualized young,
the thoughts fly unhinged.
They say that children are easy
and adults can always make the win.

MONSTER BRAIN

7, 10, 11,
not even legal in Asia.
Pre-pubescent underage,
I'd rather have phallic aplasia.

Thoughts are thoughts
not thought-fused action;
god won't judge me for
resisting the distraction.

Why isn't there therapy
for those who really do suffer
with pedophile's lust,
who see not the pants of the other?

Before desire turns action
let them get help.
Seek to change the wired brain
and turn from the porno whelp.

My soul isn't damned
for thoughts that aren't mine.
I know my brain is to blame
not my conscious mind.

Daniel Cureton

THE HAND WASHER

A one Scene play

[Curtain]

HAND WASHER *sits in a circle with a group and counselor. The chairs are undulating up and down at random as voices are heard. They are in an office discussing their problems all at once in a cacophony when* HAND WASHER's *dialogue breaks through.* OBSESSIVE COMPULSIVE DISORDER THERAPY GROUP *quiets.*
Chairs stop undulating when HAND WASHER *speaks.*
Solitary light on HAND WASHER, *others in darkness.*

HAND WASHER: Come on, I said hurry up!' is what I told my son. I'm such a hypocrite!

> [Orange lights light up behind the group member's heads. Orange lights turn off after speaking. Continue each time the group speaks.]

MONSTER BRAIN

OBSESSIVE COMPULSIVE DISORDER THERAPY GROUP (OCDTG): No, you're just struggling.

HAND WASHER: But it's horrible that I can see him doing what I do and tell him to be done, yet I can' break myself from the hand washing.

> OCDTG *Collective sigh.*
> OCDTG *Member sits pondering before asking question.*

OCDTG MEMBER: Why not set an egg timer? Instead of 15 minutes at the sink, try 10, or 5 on the timer?

HAND WASHER: It's just…it's just I can't help it. I spend so much time washing my hands and, in the shower, —that's worse—I don't know why I can't convince myself, why that after 10 minutes I'm done.

> [COUNSELOR's *mouth is illuminated by single light when they speak.*]

COUNSELOR: Logic and reason don't work. We can't reason and rationalize ourselves out of the compulsion traps when we are in OCD.

HAND WASHER: How long do you all take to wash hands??

Daniel Cureton

OCDTG MEMBER: Now, most people max will be 10 seconds: Wet, soap, rinse. Very few do 25 or more in very hot water like recommend.

    HAND WASHER *experiences Mild shock—nervous anticipation—among intermittent* OCDTG *conversation.*

OCDTG: Well, we hope you'll try. Is that a goal you want to work on for the next two weeks?

HAND WASHER: Yeah, Idk if I can do the egg timers but I recognize what I'm doing.

OCDTG MEMBER: Well, it's important you try, just live the fear. Do the exposure therapy slowly like I did with the kitchen knives and my roommate.

HAND WASHER OCD BRAIN: (*Voice over of* HAND WASHER, *sigh.*) See, see how much better you are than all the rest. Every minute ensures your family will not die of a disease you brought home, a disease you cooked into their food or gave them when you hugged them goodnight. You're gonna kill them all if you don't keep washing! You KNOW it, You FEEL it!

    Group goes back to cacophony, undulating.

MONSTER BRAIN

HAND WASHER *retreats into darkness.*

[Curtain.]

Daniel Cureton

THE SILENT SUFFERERS

(» » » = *new stanza*)

You sit on the throne,
squeezing out a turd
the only real solitude left
your family always heard
» » »
The thought strikes, "just smother them in their sleep,
It'll feel *so* good,
and the quiet hours you'll keep
you know you should."
» » »
Anxiety STINGS,

you know why it happened

intrusive persuasion on peaceful shit

and a little more MADDENED

» » »
Yet still,
let it play and pass.
You know the drill—
With a mental fast—
exposure therapy,
the only way to conquer OCD's ass.

MONSTER BRAIN

» » »

They call us **THE SILENT SUFFERERS**.
Those plagued with unwanted thoughts,
that come into mind,
TIME after TIME

» » »

Kill, suck, germ, death,
Water, handwash, pull, pick
Walk, fold, check,
and stick.

» » »

It's all in our heads.
The compulsion's way—
it's not "right," better
listen, and

"DO IT MY WAY, AS I SAY"

» » »

The mind demands we perform
ridiculous stunts
and hoaxes against ourselves
to feel complete, quiet again
or take the full brunt.

» » »

Little did we know—
 the beast, that's what's best—
Don't give in, it's always a test.

» » »

We sit in silence
performing a complex ritual
If it doesn't play out as it should
we feel as if we'll come apart, perpetual

Daniel Cureton

»»»
The end of the day brings exhaustion
as we sat and fought inside

thoughts attacking **Over** and **Over**
never relenting, never sleeping—never aside.
»»»
We let down our guard
and one little image slipped through.
Slicing your child's neck
and calling it truth.
»»»

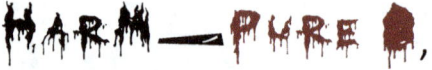

Disease will kill us (it tells us),

and **GERMS** plague our family.

HANDWASHING and

only a few types we've learned

CHECKING (*That Damned Lock*)

gives 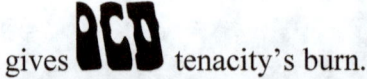 tenacity's burn.

MONSTER BRAIN

» » »

Biological mechanism, faltered 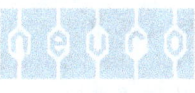 signals,

forms that 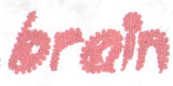 the mind.

Unconscious and **unwired**

Better sought, psychopomp's pyre.

» » »

Such horror that corrupts the *brain*

Conjures up images, fuck!
Little did you know
I suffer, and I am stuck.
» » »
It **NEVER TURNS OFF**.

Therapy helps bolster will.

LOGIC AND REASON—no shield defense,

fulcrum of anxiety's biting pills.
» » »
The mind doesn't make *sense*

We are distracted by the RITUAL

That brings temporary relief for a *minute*

Compulsion for the conscious miserable.

Daniel Cureton

»»»
Thought-fused action,
The brain tricks us with its roll.
When we believe the act,

next turn we'll LOOSE control.
»»»
WEAK inside, no turning back.

you can't see our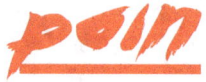

empathy's light leaves for

those without bane.
»»»
There are no signs,
only our mood.
If you could fall into our mind
you would cry too.
»»»
carriers of the BUCKETS of shame

Lifeguards at the pools of tears

bearers in the OCEAN'S tide of despair,

As we seek the SAILBOAT of hope

ever drawing near.

MONSTER BRAIN

>> >> >>

Only when we *sleep* (not even then sometimes)

are we really ourselves, true.

Let **DREAMLAND** come,

Go to the flowered fields and be free, renewed.

Daniel Cureton

HUE OF BLUE

With hue of blue, Clonazepam.
You sit on the shelf each night
eyeing me with your tranquil plot,
I resist like I know I ought.
But, can't help to think you're right.

You land inside so easily.
Taking you is so breezily.
I close my eyes before the ride,
With hue of blue.

Sleep comes as the fairy dreamland.
No better feeling than dreamsands.
I, in wake of anxiety,
escape OCD quietly.
O, there in sleep I make my stand

with hue of blue.

MONSTER BRAIN

THROUGH FIRE, AND WATER

"Go back to the SHADOW!"

"From the lowest dungeon to the highest peak, I fought with the Balrog of Morgoth. *Until at last, I threw down my enemy and smote his ruin upon the mountain side. Darkness took me, and I strayed out of thought and time. Stars wheeled overhead and everyday was as long as a life age of the Earth. But it was not the end. I felt life in me again*" (Boyens, 59-60).

"From the lowest dungeon to the highest peak...*I threw down my enemy, and he fell from the high place and broke the mountain-side where he smote it in his ruin*...Then darkness took me, and I strayed out of thought and time...while the stars wheeled over, and each day was as long as a life-age of the earth" (Tolkien, 330 and 502).

Daniel Cureton

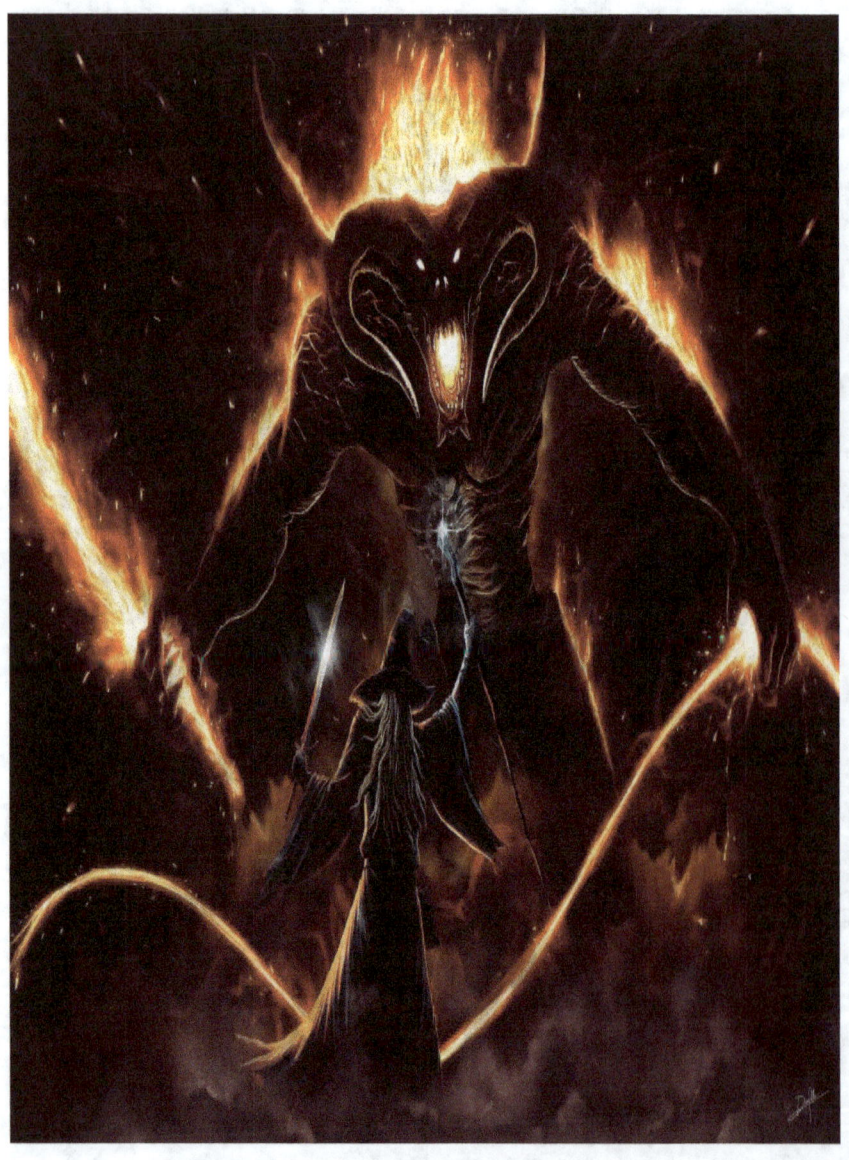

"Gandalf vs Balrog [Durin's Bane]" at the bridge of Khazad-dûm (Pilla).

Used with the permission of the artist.

I BID ADIEU

And so ends the life of self, 33 years, and begins a new person. A new journey awaits, filled with wondrous tales, poems, and friendships.

To my old self, I bid adieu:

"So long, and thanks for all the fish" (Douglas, 164).

The Lark
From "A Farewell to Saint Petersburg" (No. 10)

Daniel Cureton

Mikhail Glinka
1804 - 1857

Arr. for piano by
Mily Balakirew

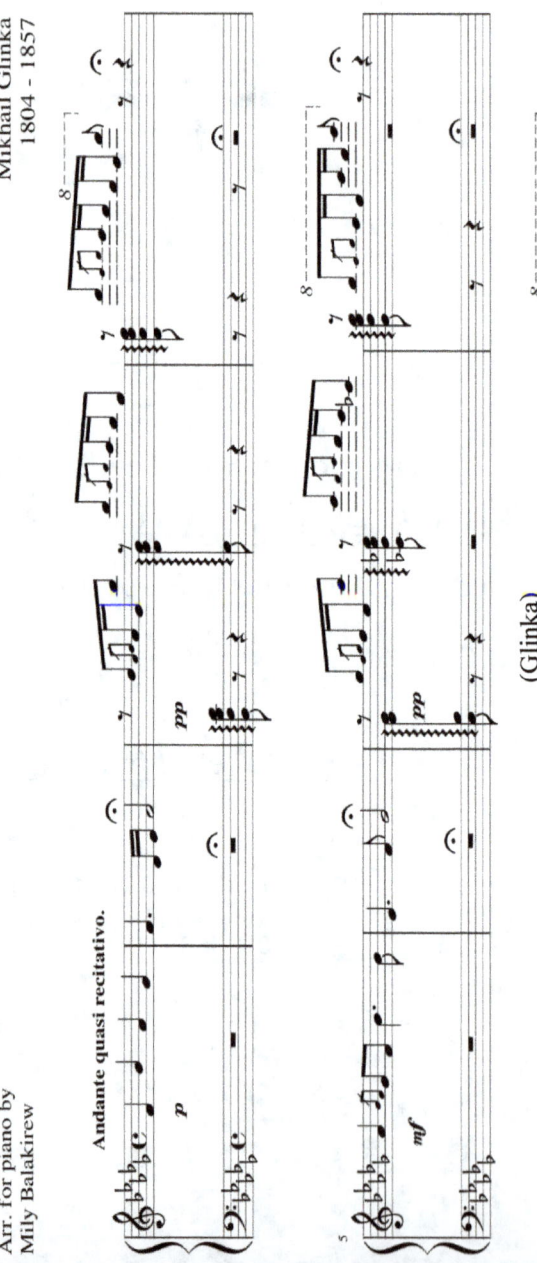

(Glinka)

MONSTER BRAIN

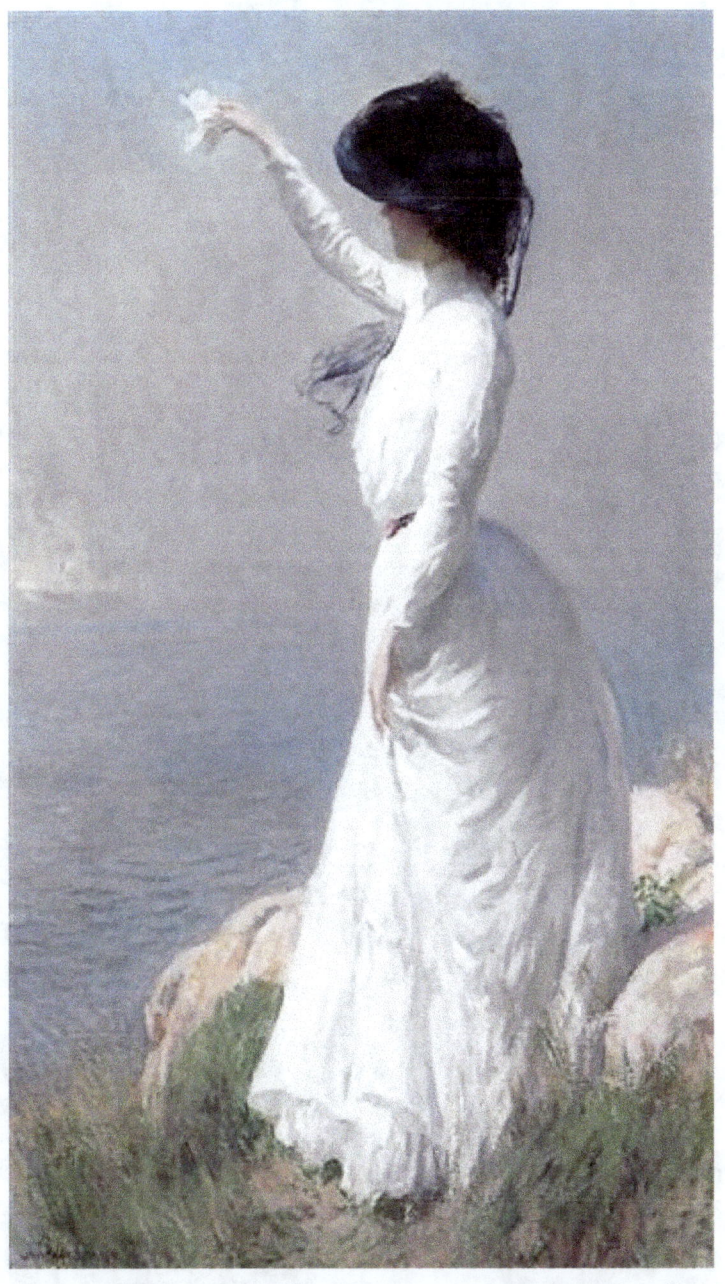

"Farewell." 1900-1902, oil on canvas (Decamp).

BIBLIOGRAPHY

Works Cited

Literary

Adams, Douglas. *The Hitchhikers' Guide to the Galaxy*. Hanomag, 2001.

Boyens, Philippa et. al. *The Lord of the Rings: The Two Towers*. New Line Cinema, 2002, https://www.raindance.org/scripts/lotr-the-two-towers.pdf. Accessed 1 Oct, 2019.

Cureton, Daniel. *Monster Brain: Conversations with OCD*. Forty-Two Books, 2019.

Trilingual Compendium of Texts. "Diagram of the Human Brain with Five Cells or Ventriculi Representing the Five 'Powers' of Thought (the Common or Imaging Sense, Imagination, Estimation, Cogitation and Memory), Illustrating Qualiter Caput Hominis Situatur." Circa 14th Century. Cambridge University Library, Cambridge, MS Gg 1.1, p. 490v, https://cudl.lib.cam.ac.uk/view/MS-GG-00001-00001/988. Accessed 1 Aug, 2019. Reproduced by kind permission of the Syndics of Cambridge University Library.

Erasmus, Desiderius Roterodamus. *The Essential Rasmus.* Translated by John P. Dolan. Mentor Book, 1964.

Tolkein, J. R. R. *The Lord of the Rings*. Houghton Mifflin Harcourt, 2004.

Video

Snape Quote

Epic Scenes. "Professor Snape and the Occlumency Lessons | Harry Potter 5 and the Order of the Phoenix 2007 HD." *Youtube*, uploaded 20 Jun, 2018, https://www.youtube.com/watch?v=V4hTVanqtBY.

Music

<u>*Public Domain*</u>

Debussy, Claude. "Images I L105 and II L105, No. 4 Cloches à Travers les Feuilles." Durand et Fils, 1908.

Glinka, Mikhail. "Glinka—The Lark from 'A Farewell to Saint Petersburg' (No. 10)." 1840. *Musescore*, uploaded by hmnscomp, 18 Oct, 2016. https://musescore.com/hmscomp/scores/2781271. Accessed 1 Aug, 2019.

Art

<u>*Public Domain*</u>

Decamp, Joseph. "Farewell." 1902, William Young and Co. USA. Online at: *Wikiart*, https://www.wikiart.org/en/joseph-decamp/farewell-1902. 1 Dec, 2016. Accessed 1 Aug, 2019.

MONSTER BRAIN

Images

Free Commercial usage

Max Pixel. "Weird scary creepy horror pumpkin fear Halloween." https://www.maxpixel.net/Weird-Scary-Creepy-Horror-Pumpkin-Fear-Halloween-2393827. Accessed 1 Aug, 2019.

Killscreen303. "Using MAME to Warp to Level 256, the split screen is shown." *Map 256 Glitch*, Pac-Man Wiki, https://pacman.fandom.com/wiki/Map_256_Glitch?file=Splitscreen.gif. Accessed 1 Aug, 2019.

K, Pablo. "Affect! Biopolitics! Technology!: A Call for Papers." The Disorder of Things, 16 Dec, 2011, https://thedisorderofthings.files.wordpress.com/2011/12/medieval-brain-map2.jpg. Accessed 1 Aug, 2019.

Brathwaite, Les Fabian. "Photos for Photos: 18 Times Jesus was the Savior of Sexiness." *Queerty,* 5 April, 2015. Q Digital, https://www.queerty.com/photos-sacrilege-18-times-jesus-was-the-savior-of-sexiness-20150405/13-63.

TheDragonLord. "Gandalf Vs Balrog.jpg." *The One Wiki to Rule Them All*, 6 Jan, 2013. Fandom, https://lotr.fandom.com/wiki/File:GandalfVSBalrog.jpg

Licensed Commercial Usage

Kapitosh. "Boom isolated white comic text speech bubble. Colored pop art style sound effect. Halftone vector illustration banner. Vintage comics book poster. Colored funny cloud font—Vector." *Shutterstock*, ID: 1097676998, https://www.shutterstock.com/image-vector/boom-isolated-white-comic-text-speech-1097676998. Accessed 1 Aug, 2019.

Fisher, Tim. "How to Fix a Blue Screen of Death: The Blue Screen of Death is Real—but Definitely Fixable." *Windows*, Lifewire, 1 July, 2019, https://www.lifewire.com/how-to-fix-a-blue-screen-of-death-2624518. Access 1 Aug. 2019.

Pilla, Daniel. "Gandalf vs Balrog." 2015. *Reddit*, posted by Lol33ta, Oct, 2018, https://www.reddit.com/r/ImaginaryMiddleEarth/comments/9odll6/gandalf_vs_balrog_by_daniel_pilla/.

It is assumed the following image is free for commercial use due to the original source URL on Tumblr being deleted.

Bee, Victoria. "OCD Awareness Ribbon, OCD Fighter." *Pinterest*, https://www.pinterest.com/pin/355925176780517409/. Accessed 1 Sept, 2019.

Fonts

Licensed Commercial Usage

Andrade, Phillip G. "Nasal Drip." *Dafont,* 11 Aug. 2005. Dry Heaves Fonts: 2015, https://www.dafont.com/nasal-drip.font. Accessed 1 Aug, 2019.

Blake, Stephenson. "French Script MT." Inland Type Foundry, 1905. Monotype Type Drawing Office, 1989, https://docs.microsoft.com/en-us/typography/font-list/french-script-mt. Accessed 1 Aug. 2019.

MONSTER BRAIN

Dies. "Tesla." *Dafont*, 11 Jan, 2017, https://www.dafont.com/tesla.font. Accessed 1 Aug. 2019.

Clark, Curtis. "Elder Futhark." *Dafont*. Mockfont: 1998, https://www.dafont.com/elder-futhark.font. Accessed 1 Aug, 2019.

Harris, Jonathan S. "Asylum Mansion." *Dafont*, 9 Apr, 2014, https://www.dafont.com/jonathan-s-harris.d3456. Accessed 1 Aug, 2019.

—. "Silly People." *Dafont,* 23 Dec, 2012, https://www.dafont.com/silly-people.font. Accessed 1 Aug, 2019.

—. "Your Bloody Choice." *Dafont*, 4 Oct, 2012, https://www.dafont.com/your-bloody-choice.font. Accessed 1 Aug, 2019.

Kerkhoff, David. "Skratch." *Dafont,* 24 Nov, 2010. Hand of Fonts, https://www.dafont.com/skratch.font. Accessed 1 Aug, 2019.

Misti. "Mf This is Ridiculous." *Dafont*, 25 Nov, 2013. Misti's Fonts, https://www.dafont.com/this-is-ridiculous.font. Accessed 1 Aug, 2019.

Nelson, Brad. "Bubleman." *Brain Eaters Font Co.* 1001 Fonts, https://www.1001fonts.com/bubble-man-font.html. Accessed 1 Aug, 2019.

Morison, Stanley. "Times New Roman." *The Times,* 1931, https://docs.microsoft.com/en-us/typography/font-list/times-new-roman. Accessed 1 Aug, 2019.

Daniel Cureton

Nikolic, Vladimir. "Cosmology." *Dafont*, 10 Jan, 2018, https://www.dafont.com/cosmology.font. Accessed 1 Aug, 2019.

Steinok, Dan. "Sailor Scrawl Fancy." *Dafont*, 4 Oct, 2013. Out of Step Font Company, https://www.dafont.com/sailor-scrawl.font. Accessed 1 Aug, 2019.

The Crow is Mine. "Psyche Ward." *Font Space,* 16 Apr, 2019. The Crow is Mine, 2019, https://www.fontspace.com/thecrownismine/psyche-ward. Accessed 1 Aug, 2019.

Ydhra Studio. "Boatman." *Dafont,* 28 Sept. 2018: https://www.dafont.com/boatman.font. Accessed 1 Aug, 2019.

Zadorozny, Daniel. "Alpha Sentry." *Urban Fonts*. Iconian Fonts, 2007, https://www.dafont.com/alpha-sentry.font. Accessed 1 Aug, 2019.

—. "Byte Police 3D." *Free Fonts*, Nov 2018. Iconian Fonts, 2007, https://www.ffonts.net/Byte-Police-3D.font. Accessed 1 Aug, 2019.

—. "Charlie's Angles Outgradient." *Urban Fonts*. Iconian Fonts, 2007, https://www.urbanfonts.com/fonts/Charlie_s_Angles.font. Accessed 1 Aug, 2019.

—. "Frozen Crystal." *Dafont,* 26 June, 2016. Iconian Fonts, 2007, https://www.dafont.com/iconian-fonts.d6. Accessed 1 Aug, 2019.

—. "Pocket Monster Leaftalic." *Dafont,* 23 Oct, 2016. Iconian Fonts, 2007, https://www.dafont.com/pocket-monster.font. Accessed 1 Aug, 2019.

<u>*Free Commercial Usage*</u>

Bonislawsky, Brian J. "Rocky." *Dafont,* 20 Oct, 2006. Astigmatic One Eye Typographic Institute, https://www.dafont.com/rocky.font. Accessed 1 Aug, 2019.

Curtis, Nick. "Lost Wages." *Dafont*. Nick's Fonts, https://www.dafont.com/lost-wages.font. Accessed 1 Aug, 2019.

KA Fonts. "KASnake." *Fontspace*, 30 Apr, 2010. KA Fonts, 1993, https://www.fontspace.com/ka-fonts/kasnake. Accessed 1 Aug, 2019.

Larabie, Ray. "Welfare Brat." *Dafont,* 18 June, 2012. Typodermic Fonts, https://www.dafont.com/welfare-brat.font. Accessed 1 Aug, 2019.

Murphy, Tom. "Germs." *Dafont,* 22 July, 2007. Divide by Zero, 23 July, 1996, https://www.dafont.com/germs.font. Accessed 1 Aug, 2019.

Steffman Dieter. "Flowers Initials." *1001 Fonts*. Tyopgrapher Mediengestaltung, https://www.1001fonts.com/flowers-initials-font.html#styles. Accessed 1 Aug, 2019.

It is assumed the following fonts are free for commercial use as the owners are not able to be contacted in any form.

Gauthier, John. "A Quiet Sleep." *Dafont*, 18 Feb, 2015, https://www.dafont.com/a-quiet-sleep.font. Accessed 1 Aug, 2019.

Mueller, Richard William. "Meltdown MF." *Dafont,* 17 Oct, 2005, https://www.dafont.com/meltdown-mf.font. Accessed 1 Aug, 2019.

"Ravie." *Font Zone*, https://fontzone.net/font-details/ravie. Accessed 1 Aug, 2019.

Schizoid, Nihilist. "Homicide Effect." *Dafont,* 24 July, 2006, https://www.dafont.com/homicide-effect.font. Accessed 1 Aug, 2019.

Ziehn, Jens R. "Monster AG." *1001 Free Fonts*. Film Himmel, https://www.1001freefonts.com/monster-ag.font. Accessed 22 Sept, 2019.

References

Introduction

Editors. "Obsessive-Compulsive Disorder." *Psychology*, 12 Oct, 2017, Encyclopedia Britannica, 20 July, 1998, https://www.britannica.com/science/obsessive-compulsive-disorder. Accessed 22 Sept, 2019.

Hershfield, Jon et. al. *Everyday Mindfulness for OCD: Tips, Tricks, and Skills for Living Joyfully*. New Harbinger Publications, 2017.

Hershfield, Jon and Grayson, Jonathan. *Overcoming Harm OCD: Mindfulness and CBT Tools for Coping with Unwanted Violent Thoughts*. New Harbinger Publications, 2018.

Goldenberg, Michael. *Harry Potter and the Order of the Phoenix.* Warner Bros. Pictures, 2007, p. 109, http://www.dailyscript.com/scripts/HARRY-POTTER-AND-THE-ORDER-OF-THE-PHOENIX-2007-by-Michael-Goldenberg.pdf. Accessed 1 Oct, 2019.

Some Stirring Passages

Rushdie, Salman. *The Satanic Verses*. The Viking Press, 1989.

The Conversations

Golding, William. *Lord of the Flies*. Faber and Faber, 1954.

Shakespeare, William. *The Taming of the Shrew*. London, Peter Shortand, 1594, https://shakespearedocumented.folger.edu/file/69594-title-page

Music

Beatles. "All You Need is Love." *1 Remixed/Remastered*, Capitol, 2015.

YOGI, MC. "Krishna Dub (Remix)." *Elephant Power*, White Swan, 2008.

ABOUT THE AUTHOR

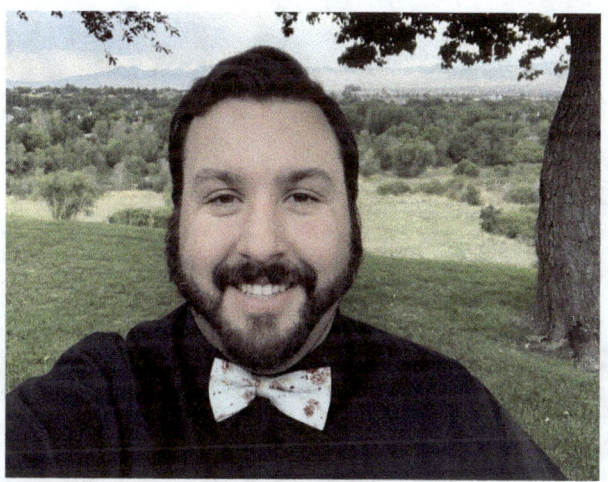

Daniel is a writer, editor, publisher, and avant-garde poet. His poetry exposes the deeper meanings of experiential living and his stories are idea platforms. He holds an MA in English from Weber State University.

Originally from South Carolina, Daniel currently lives in Salt Lake City, UT with his cat Oliver, a cross eyed Siamese.

Notes

www.ingramcontent.com/pod-product-compliance
Lightning Source LLC
Chambersburg PA
CBHW052035070526
44584CB00016B/2054